'In *Self Psychology: Moving from Theory to Practice*, Jill Gardner, a superlative teacher, helps both the psychoanalytic beginner and the seasoned therapist to understand Self Psychology, one of the most important theories/practices in recent psychoanalysis. She does not choose between theory and practice, but shows how they stimulate and enrich each other. Her inviting writing helps the reader to embrace essential lifelong learning. I love this book.'

Donna M. Orange, *PhD, PsyD, faculty, NYU postdoc and the Institute for the Psychoanalytic Study of Subjectivity, New York*

'Jill Gardner has written a superbly lucid volume that brings the therapist into the consulting room and addresses the needs of clinicians who struggle to integrate theory with clinical practice. Demonstrating masterful understanding, this accessible and wonderful book is also a valuable resource for supervisors and teachers as it traces the history of Self Psychology's healing powers.'

Richard A. Geist, *EdD, Massachusetts Institute for Psychoanalysis; clinical instructor part-time Emeritus, Harvard Medical School*

'Endorsing Jill Gardner's new book, *Self Psychology: Moving from Theory to Practice*, fills me with pride and pleasure. I am amazed at the clarity and depth of her understanding of the clinical process, and I am certain that clinicians, whether experienced or novice, will profit greatly from reading Jill Gardner's new contribution.'

Estelle Shane, *PhD, faculty, and training and supervising analyst, at The Institute for Contemporary Psychoanalysis and The New Center for Psychoanalysis, Los Angeles*

Self Psychology

This book offers an in-depth explanation of the concepts of self psychology and pragmatic steps for recognizing and using these concepts in clinical work, helping clinicians move from theory to practice.

Both early and contemporary concepts in self psychology and inter-subjectivity theory are discussed in successive chapters of the book, with illustrative examples drawn from the author's experience working in diverse settings with a wide range of mental health practitioners. Individual chapters shed light on brief treatment, supervision, interpretation, development, agency and nuances of empathic communication, among other topics. In addressing these topics, specific tools for conceptualizing clinical data and guidelines for intervention are also described. The emphasis on helping people via a sustained focus on their internal, subjective experience and creating a new selfobject bond with the therapist unifies the chapters in this volume.

With its rich clinical vignettes and accessible language, *Self Psychology: Moving from Theory to Practice* is also a valuable resource for supervisors and teachers of self psychology, whether in analytic training institutes, graduate schools of psychology, counseling and social work or continuing education programs.

Jill R. Gardner, PhD, is a clinical psychologist in private practice in Chicago, Illinois, where she has also served as lecturer and professional development program faculty at the University of Chicago.

NEW DIRECTIONS IN SELF PSYCHOLOGY BOOK SERIES
GEORGE HAGMAN
Series Editor

Since Heinz Kohut's *The Analysis of the Self* was published in 1971, psychoanalytic Self Psychology has developed into a theory and mode of treatment which is complex and multi-dimensional as well as vital and still evolving. Enlisting authors from a variety of disciplines, and under the editorship of psychoanalyst and social worker George Hagman, the *New Directions in Self Psychology: Clinical, Research and Cultural Applications* book series will examine the state-of-the-art in Self Psychology, providing an opportunity for authors to explore and extend the model in new directions.

Once limited to a small group centered in Chicago, Self Psychology currently has adherent organizations on every continent. Over the past half century, Self Psychology has influenced academic disciplines such as history, political science, art history and social theory, as well as psychological research into child development, neuropsychology, addiction and psychopathology. Its influence on psychotherapy has been enormous, with many analytic and non-analytic models benefiting from its concepts such as motivational interviewing, grief therapies, addiction treatments and person-centered counseling. Most importantly, Self Psychology has continued to thrive in the field of psychoanalysis, being elaborated and augmented by the contribution of many subspecialties such as motivational systems theory, intersubjectivity theory, relational psychoanalysis, systems theory and complexity.

The volumes in this series will be devoted to a variety of topics including, but not limited to, couples' treatment, addiction, depression and bereavement, intersubjective Self Psychology, adolescence, infant research, Relational Self Psychology, culture and historical theory. Specific clinical subjects will be highlighted such as the selfobject transference, rethinking resistance, new understandings of empathy, neuro-psychoanalysis, relationality, trauma and grief. The editor invites contributions from across these areas of practice and the subject areas previously mentioned toward the promotion of a vital culture of debate and experimentation in the field of Self Psychology.

For more information about this series, please visit: https://www.routledge.com/New-Directions-in-Self-Psychology/book-series/NDSP.

Kohut's Self Psychology for a Fractured World
New Ways of Understanding the Self and Human Community
John Riker

Self Psychology

Moving from Theory to Practice

Jill R. Gardner, PhD

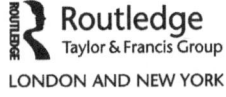
Routledge
Taylor & Francis Group

LONDON AND NEW YORK

Designed cover image: © Getty Images

First published 2025
by Routledge
4 Park Square, Milton Park, Abingdon, Oxon OX14 4RN

and by Routledge
605 Third Avenue, New York, NY 10158

Routledge is an imprint of the Taylor & Francis Group, an informa business

British Library Cataloguing-in-Publication Data
A catalogue record for this book is available from the British Library

ISBN: 9781032793122 (hbk)
ISBN: 9781032793115 (pbk)
ISBN: 9781003491453 (ebk)

DOI: 10.4324/9781003491453

Typeset in Times New Roman
by KnowledgeWorks Global Ltd.

for Miriam Elson

Contents

Foreword

I am proud to preface this book by Jill Gardner, PhD, *Self Psychology: Moving from Theory to Practice*, which is Volume 2 of the book series "New Directions in Self Psychology." For many years, Jill has been a fellow member, leader, friend and teacher within the community of Self Psychology. Jill's good cheer, warmth and selflessness have made her a beloved colleague to many of us, contributing in innumerable ways to the communities within which she has lived and worked.

"New Directions in Self Psychology" was created as a showcase for new voices and selected senior ones which, by organizing their ideas into book form, brings together the best of each author's thoughts in an integrated and accessible form. In this volume, Jill has gathered together her major contributions to Self Psychology and to mental health practitioners in all disciplines. She does so through a group of essays which capture and convey the ideas of Self Psychology in a manner that is straightforward, clear and understandable to clinicians at any level of knowledge and expertise. Her grasp of psychoanalytic ideas is clear and practical. She demystifies psychoanalytic self psychology, providing guidance regarding how to be and what to do as a therapist, while showing how the concepts of Self Psychology can help make sense of a wide variety of clinical challenges.

Jill's knowledge and skills were forged in diverse clinical and educational settings. For 20 years she was a therapist, supervisor and administrator at a Community Mental Health Center in Chicago. It was during this time that she encountered Self Psychology and recognized the theory's potential utility for diverse patients, clinical conditions and practice settings. Although she was herself a psychologist trained in and practicing long-term psychoanalytic psychotherapy, at the mental health center she developed a model of short-term treatment anchored in the theory of Self Psychology.

For 15 years she also taught graduate courses in Self Psychology at the University of Chicago's Crown Family School of Social Work, Policy, and Practice, as well as continuing education workshops there, at the Chicago Psychoanalytic Institute and at multiple community agencies and clinics.

Most importantly, Jill has been a beloved supervisor and a teacher of supervisors for many years. Her application of Self Psychology to supervision has been invaluable to many, and her faith in the supervisory relationship as an avenue to professional development is grounded in extensive experience with clinicians working in a wide-ranging array of settings.

As Jill shares some of her wisdom in the chapters of this book, she conveys concepts and clinical approaches in a sensible and useful manner that the reader will find enlightening and refreshing. A compliment that I made to Jill after one of her many talks was that she embodies psychoanalysis for the common therapist: clear, straightforward and without artifice. So, you will find in this book a distillation of the best of Jill Gardner the therapist and person, and we as readers can now reap the benefits of learning from such a special clinician and teacher.

George Hagman, LCSW
Editor, New Directions in Self Psychology Book Series

Acknowledgements

I never expected to teach at the University of Chicago, give a Kohut Memorial Lecture or write a book. These things and many others happened because I had the immense good fortune to be blessed with opportunity, guidance, encouragement and support from so many individuals along the way. Recognizing them all feels like it would take longer than the book, but I want to name more than a few.

Opportunity begins with my mother, Eileen Gardner, who wanted her daughter to have the opportunity she never did to have an education and a vocation and who steadfastly guarded my chance to do both. Enormously articulate herself, she always urged me to speak with clarity. My path was equally influenced by my father, Leon Gardner, from whom I inherited a capacity to break down complex things into their component parts and who took great joy himself in explaining, teaching and empowering others, whether it was to help someone improve their tennis shot or show me how to work the soda fountain in his drug store. I am grateful for the gift of my parents being who they were in these ways that gave me so much.

Madeline Gomez, the medical director of the community mental health center where I started my career, welcomed my introduction of self psychology into our short-term treatment model. Looking back, I appreciate the multiple ways her affirming presence facilitated my professional growth.

Virtually every chapter in this book was written with material developed first in response to invitations to present or teach. My thanks start with Karen Teigiser, who first invited me to teach professional development seminars in self psychology, and later graduate courses, at the University of Chicago. I am also grateful for the opportunity Annette Richard gave me to present a day-long workshop in Montreal and similar invitations from Eldad Idan in Jerusalem and from Amanda Kottler and Kim de la Harpe in Cape Town to meet with their local self psychology groups. I am thankful to Shelley Doctors for her invitation to present a Kohut Memorial Lecture and her warm introduction of me when I did, along with Brenda Solomon's endorsement to take it on. I also particularly value Ernest Wolfe's invitation to teach with him on Cape Cod and in Dreieich, Germany. Through each of these opportunities, I further developed the ideas found in this book.

I am eternally grateful for the inestimable contribution of my mentor, Miriam Elson, whom I describe in greater detail in Chapter 9. Miriam guided my learning, encouraged me to write and helped to edit my initial efforts. Helpful suggestions on other writings in this book have come from Ann Bergart, Diana Beliard, Carla Leone, Anna Ornstein, Donna Orange, Dick Geist and Dan Perlitz, among others.

I was fortunate to come of age in self psychology at a time and place that allowed me to know personally many of Kohut's close collaborators, including Marian Tolpin, Arnold Goldberg, Paul and Anna Ornstein, Michael Basch and Ernie Wolfe. I am grateful for their brilliant writings, their friendship, and their guidance and support.

Encouragement and support have come from a multitude of others as well: from Bill Borden, with whom I co-taught advanced psychodynamic practice and whose friendship and keen intellect have always enriched me; from Diana Lidofsky, who affirmed the value of my written work for others by using it in teaching her medical residents; from Eldad Idan and Donna Orange, who have always been so affirming of my efforts; and from George Hagman, whose warm invitation and encouragement were the impetus for writing this book and without whom it would surely not exist. I deeply appreciate them all.

In a category of his own is my analyst, Paul Tolpin. Nothing enabled me to understand self psychology as much as the experience of being his patient. I am grateful for all the ways he helped me, both personally and professionally, to become who I am.

Since the beginning of the pandemic, I have been very actively involved in three groups of colleagues. In my incredible peer supervision/consultation group, Amanda Kottler, Dan Perlitz, Annette Richard, Joye Weisel-Barth and I, experienced therapists all, consistently present our most difficult clinical challenges and invariably gain extraordinary new insights and help from each other.

When the International Association of Psychoanalytic Self Psychology formed Covid support groups at the start of the pandemic, I was lucky to land in one that included Doris Brothers, Dan Perlitz, Annette Richard,

Jon Sletvold, Margy Sperry and Judy Zevon. These colleagues have offered not only support and friendship, but wonderful opportunities for dialogue about our work and other issues important to us all.

Finally, I am inspired by what I call my developing-ideas-about-therapeutic-process group, which includes Christina Connell, Dan Perlitz, Estelle Shane and, keeping us all on track, Kathy Wetmore. In this group we have been working together to develop training materials integrating theory and practice, which we are road-testing in workshops at our conference. Thinking and drafting materials together has involved great synergy, creative ideas and a lot of laughter.

All of these wonderful colleagues, most of whom I met with weekly, have offered support, encouragement, stimulating ideas and deepening friendships, for which I am deeply appreciative.

Closer to home, I have participated for many years with colleagues in the Midwest Self Psychology Study Group. Very recently we've added many new members, but the ones I have been meeting with for a very long time and who have greatly contributed to and enriched my understanding of the ideas in this book include Karen Bloomberg, Lynn Borenstein, Denise Davis, Scott Davis, Marcia Dobson, Gail Elden, Amy Eldridge, Elizabeth Feldman, Jim Fisch, Lucy Freund, Carla Leone, Karen Martin, Shelly Meyers, Gavin Mullen, John Riker, Allen Siegel, Brenda Solomon, David Solomon, Jeffrey Stern, David Terman, Jeanne Walbridge, Neurine Wiggin and Molly Wittin. I am grateful for their insights and their openness in sharing their own work, deepening my understanding of multiple perspectives.

One of the study groups that I lead myself, mostly comprised of former supervisees, has been meeting for nearly 35 years, with almost entirely the same membership. Diana Beliard, Leigh Chethik, Betty Contorer, David Fireman, Carla Leone, Diana Mercer and Rick Volden have opened their lives, their minds and their clinical practice to each other and to me with an intimacy and depth that have enhanced us all. They have been a stimulus to formulate and express my own ideas clearly, and I am deeply grateful for their friendship.

The members of my other study group, some of whom have been with me nearly as long, have likewise shared their clinical work and ideas with each other and with me in ways that continue to add to my own growth along with theirs. For this I am thankful to Erin Ader, Karuna Bahadur, Gail Elden, Kathy Kesselring, Christina Peters, Jeanne Pozy, Mary Sayers, Amy Schiller, Carrie Torgerson and Alina Viola.

In addition to all these people I have named, there are countless unnamed others—the patients who have given me the honor of entrusting the intimate story of their lives with me and the supervisees, students and workshop attendees who have, by their questions, reactions and challenges, helped me understand how to be helpful and how to improve my ability both to teach and to treat. It is more than a truism that we grow at least as much by doing and teaching as by being taught. I am similarly grateful to those patients, supervisees and students who have given me permission to share aspects of their own lives and our work in clinical examples that I've included in this volume.

We all live in an intersubjective world, where our experience is co-determined by the people and context within which we find ourselves. I have the ability to write this book because, and only because, of the enormous contribution of all the people I've just described. Every variant of nourishing selfobject experience *vis-à-vis* idealizing, mirroring and twinship is evident in the professional relationships I've been fortunate to have in my life. I am deeply grateful for them all. And I am grateful for Heinz Kohut, for his breaking the new ground that has provided us all with such powerful ideas and concepts for doing our work.

Writing a book, even with many parts drawn from earlier writings, is a time-consuming endeavor. I am grateful for the forbearance of my spouse, Merle Shapera, in supporting without complaint the countless hours I've spent squirreled away in my office. Also, as my first reader, Merle's editorial suggestions inevitably steer me away from pitfalls and make my prose better. But most of all, I deeply appreciate her endless encouragement, enjoyment and pride in my efforts, and her enduring love.

To those who have read this far, I want to say that I hope you enjoy this book and I hope you find it helpful. I am grateful for the opportunity to offer to others even a portion of what I've been so abundantly given by all the people I've just acknowledged.

For granting permission to include in this volume the following, previously published article authored by me, I am grateful to the American Psychological Association: In Chapter 2. (1991). The application of self psychology to brief psychotherapy. *Psychoanalytic Psychology, 8,* 477–500.

For granting permission to include in this volume the following, previously published articles authored by me, I am grateful to Taylor and Francis: In Chapter 3. (1999). Using self psychology in brief psychotherapy. *Psychoanalytic Social Work, 6,* 43–85; In Chapter 4. (1995).

Supervision of trainees: Tending the professional self. *Clinical Social Work Journal, 23*, 271–286; In Chapter 5. (2020). Discussion of Richard Geist's "Interpretation as carrier of selfobject functions: Catalyzing inborn potential." *Psychoanalysis, Self and Context, 15*, 348–352; In Chapter 6. 2020). Discussion of George Hagman's "Self-agency: Context and freedom in psychoanalysis." *Psychoanalysis, Self and Context, 15*, 40–46; In Chapter 7. (2021). Whither the self in Relational Self Psychology? A comment on Magid, Fosshage & Shane's article. *Psychoanalysis, Self and Context, 16*, 315–318; In Chapter 8. (2024). Forms and transformations of empathy: Subtleties and complexities of empathic communication. *Psychoanalysis, Self and Context, 19*, 80–93; In Chapter 9. (2015). Journeys and generations: Tending the professional self. *International Journal of Psychoanalytic Self Psychology, 10*, 408–420.

I also am very thankful to Routledge editor Kate Hawes, editorial assistant Aakriti Aggarwal and again George Hagman for their helpful guidance in producing this manuscript.

Introduction

There are a number of excellent introductions to self psychology already published, as well as other volumes that outline how the theory has evolved over time and how it compares with other systems of contemporary psychoanalytic thought. With so many books already available to read and study, I think any author should answer the question, "What are you hoping to contribute by adding another to all those we already have?"

My intent in this volume is both more narrow and more specific than what we find in these comprehensive introductions. I want to collect a series of articles I've written for the purpose of helping practitioners learn, teach and apply the concepts of self psychology in their clinical work, via a particular combination of theoretical exposition and clinical pragmatism.

This focus and the reason for creating this volume stem from my observation that a great many practitioners struggle to integrate their theoretical knowledge with their clinical work. After a long career of teaching, training and supervising clinicians, I've seen many people who can present clinical work vividly, but have difficulty conceptualizing what they are seeing or doing, while others seem to understand and can describe theory or concepts very well in principle, but struggle to recognize or use them clinically.

This book aims to connect theory and practice by explaining concepts in straight-forward, concrete ways and illustrating them with examples that are experience-near, familiar and common enough that clinicians can identify with them, both in their patients and in themselves. I chose the title *Self Psychology: Moving from Theory to Practice* because I wanted a title that was straight-forward—simple, direct and accessible. In this sense, it not only describes the content of the book, i.e., how to translate theory into practice, but is also emblematic of the style or process I am trying to use. This process rests on the assumption that writing doesn't have to be complex to describe and discuss complex ideas. I try to write as if talking to people, in order to make the ideas easier to understand. This means creating a path that others can follow, in language they can understand, staying linear rather than tangential and illustrating with examples that are familiar and common enough that others can readily relate to them. I chose the term "self psychology" in the title because of the emphasis I place on the enduring aspects of the theories that began with Heinz Kohut. But as the book unfolds, the increasing contributions and concepts of intersubjectivity theory and what is now called relational self psychology become increasingly evident.

Kohut was a brilliant clinician and theoretician, who gave us in self psychology a set of immensely important and powerful ideas for understanding and helping people. But, as Robert Jay Lifton said in a letter to Charles Strozier on the difficulty of reading Kohut, "to understand Kohut, he needs to be relieved of his language" (Strozier et al., 2022, p. xi). I want to provide people with a useable language for understanding and using the powerful ideas that Kohut and the many people who followed have given us.

Another aim of this book is to function as a resource for supervisors and teachers of self psychology, in both its original and contemporary forms, across diverse settings and disciplines. The chapters that follow reflect the wide applicability of self psychological ideas for different patient populations, settings and activities. Having taught mental health practitioners in a wide range of professions (physicians, nurses, psychologists, social workers and counselors), working in a wide range of practice settings (community mental health, hospital, social service agencies and private practice) and having conducted a wide range of activities besides psychotherapy (supervision, training, university teaching, management and organizational consulting), I have seen a very diverse group of people find the ideas of self psychology to be relevant and helpful in their work. So I've drawn in these chapters from a broad range of clinical examples.

This is in contrast to most of our published analytic literature, which draws its clinical examples largely from cases of psychoanalysis or intensive psychotherapy. Essential as those examples are, practitioners engaged in this wide swath of professions, settings and activities also hunger for clinical examples that more closely resemble the contexts in which they work, in language they can understand. The variety of examples offered in the chapters that follow, along with the pragmatic focus, particularly in Chapters 2, 3, 4 and 8, is intended to address this need.

The material presented in this book was developed over several decades. Over this time we have seen many changes in our concepts, our language and our ways of thinking and talking about our work. Scientific advances have helped to confirm, explain and deepen earlier ideas. For example, infant research and attachment studies have supported Kohut's conjectures about early development; the discovery of mirror neurons enhanced our understanding of the biological substrate of empathy and embeddedness; and non-linear dynamic systems and complexity theories clarified the ways neither development nor therapeutic change occurs in a single line or fixed sequence.

Both Chapter 2 and Chapter 8 start with brief summaries of theory, but this theory is cast in quite different terms, reflecting the 30+ year difference between when those chapters were first written. The earliest chapters reflect the understanding of self psychology as rendered in the 1970s and 1980s. By the last chapters, we are in a thoroughly relational, intersubjective world where the emphasis is on bi-directionality, mutual influence and co-creation of experience in the analytic relationship. Where therapeutic action is described initially in terms of structure building via the internalization of selfobject functions as self functions, it is later framed in terms of the identification, illumination and transformation of the patient's internal world, as the therapist becomes a new partner in their affective and relational experience. From ideas originally expressed largely in one-person terms, we now understand that all experience is intersubjectively constituted—organized and reorganized, formed and transformed—in specific relational contexts. Many of these changes between where we started and where we are now are reflected in the successive chapters and ideas laid out in the book.

Theory matters. It's how we organize and make sense of what we see and what we do. In an early paper on the nature and role of interpretation, Goldberg (1985) described a patient whose first analyst understood her depression in terms of oral deprivation and/or profound envy. In contrast, Goldberg believed her deficiency was not of oral supplies or of a penis, but rather was the lack of an admiring and mirroring selfobject. This difference resulted in a totally different direction and course of her treatment. Goldberg then went on to say that, "No sort of prolonged empathic immersion would reveal this material until and unless one is possessed of a theory that allows one to see it as such ... Possessed of a theory of self psychology, the psychoanalyst is a changed participant in the analytic process" (p. 64).

In a similar vein, if we believe that the absence of needed selfobject experience weakens and leaves the self vulnerable, we will try to identify the missing experiences and see how they may be sought and/or experienced in the therapeutic relationship. If we believe that the needed change is in the transformation of internal organizing principles, emotional rules or defensive strategies that are no longer needed or useful, we will try to illuminate the internal assumptions that drive the patient's experience. Either way provides some kind of roadmap for how to understand what's wrong, what's needed and what we're trying to do. But it still leaves the question of how do we do it. This is a unifying thread that runs through all the chapters. Whichever concepts we're using, we need to see how to translate them into practice.

So, in the early chapters on brief treatment I offer frameworks for determining what kind of selfobject experiences the person may have lost or missed, with detailed frameworks for assessing the state of the self. In the latter part of the book, I look at how nuances of how we communicate our empathic understanding function to identify and transform implicit assumptions and unconscious organizing principles. Both involve examples of ways to operationalize core concepts, translating theory into observable phenomena and useable guidelines for practice.

One could of course ask why we should bother with earlier conceptions that we have subsequently expanded or changed in significant ways. I think the answer lies in the fact that seeing how these earlier formulations can be helpfully translated into practice helps us understand the power and utility of ideas we don't want to lose. Rather, they become part of an expanded tapestry. Although the descriptions of therapeutic action written in 1991 and 2024 are expressed in very different terms, the utility of the latter does not cancel the utility of the former. The earlier works contain ideas that are rarely written about in quite the same detail these days. But we need those descriptions, especially for people who are learning this theory, because the early ideas are still foundational to what we do.

By way of example, if we write now in terms of illuminating and transforming internal experience, it remains no less important for people to understand the meaning of the selfobject concept in terms of its forms and transformations in healthy development and psychopathology, how it plays out with increasing complexity in the therapeutic relationship and how to identify its manifestations, presence and absence in the patient's history, current life and the treatment relationship. Chapter 3 in this book addresses how to do this in ways that more recent writings in our literature and journals no longer do.

As I looked back over the successive chapters in this book, I noticed something I hadn't realized before. Understanding the positive functions of certain seemingly dysfunctional behaviors, symptoms and defenses was always part of the theory, and these things are described as such from the first chapter on. But they would have been so much easier to describe and explain with the concept and language of the forward edge. Although Jule Miller described what Kohut meant by this term in his 1985 paper, it wasn't until Marian Tolpin resurrected the concept in 2002 that it began to take hold more widely. In the papers I wrote in the 1990s, I see it was always there implicitly. I just didn't yet know what to call it. Now it is pervasively present in the literature, and I find it to be one of the most important concepts we have in self psychology.

Having noted that changes in the evolution of our theoretical understanding and concepts over the past several decades are woven across the successive chapters that follow, I want to equally note what has *not* changed. There are abiding concepts in self psychology that from the beginning and continuing to the present are central to its enormous power and clinical utility.

Certainly, the most important of these core concepts are empathy and selfobject experience. It is no accident that when, in 2023, the organizers of the 44th annual conference of the International Association of Psychoanalytic Self Psychology wanted to plan the meeting around the cutting edge of the theory, they chose these two concepts as the topic of the first plenaries. These ideas were introduced by Kohut, subsequently developed and expanded by multiple others and continue to be understood and written about with ever increasing complexity.

It is impossible to overestimate the importance of a selfobject bond, both in development and in treatment. It is the origin and nexus of relational experience, informed by a mutual and bi-directional empathic process. I've always been struck by how Marian Tolpin described this bond. I've never seen it in print. It was, rather, something I heard her say at a professional meeting. What she said, simply but profoundly, was, "The self, supported, is a different self." For me, this simple statement captures the essence of why our therapeutic relationships are so central to the process of growth and change. I cannot count the number of times I have repeated it to trainees in order to help them understand the power of a selfobject bond. It's what

Miriam Elson likewise urged her students to understand as "the power of your presence." Finally, Strozier made a similar point when he wrote that "a troubled person in the experience of empathy becomes a different person" (Strozier et al., 2022, p. 7).

In all its forms and transformations, self psychology has retained an abiding focus on helping people via a sustained focus on their internal, subjective experience. Empathy is the means by which this inner world of another is revealed to us. Our theory is based on process rather than content. It is a methodology that stems from a certain attitude. That attitude is one of curiosity, non-judgmental inquiry and trust. It also is a theory that believes in an inherent striving toward health and growth, when the right facilitating conditions are met. These central tenets of self psychology are elaborated in the chapters that follow.

I do not distinguish between psychoanalysis and psychotherapy in this book. Rather, I see the use and translation of self psychological concepts as equally applicable regardless of the length or frequency of the treatment. The word therapist is used to refer to any practitioner, whether psychoanalyst, psychotherapist, counselor, teacher or other kind of helper. Although clinicians in varied settings may refer to the people they help as patients or clients, I generally use the term "patient," based on my own first years of practice in a hospital setting and the more customary use of this term in the bulk of the psychoanalytic literature.

The chapters of the book are divided into three parts. Part One, consisting of Chapters 1 through 4, involves writings and explication of what is often referred to as classical self psychology, using and illustrating basic concepts before the relational turn infused the self psychology literature.

Chapter 1 is a previously unpublished talk I gave as part of a panel on the treatment of personality disorders from various theoretical perspectives. My talk had to be under ten minutes, and the audience could not be assumed to know anything about self psychology. So for this purpose it was necessary to condense my words to the essence of the theory in the most parsimonious way possible. I've included it as a starting point for its value as an overview of how the essence of our theory was understood at that time.

Chapters 2 and 3 were written with the goal of establishing time-limited or brief psychotherapy as an appropriate domain for the application of self psychology and demonstrating how it could be put to use in that context. Chapter 2 offers a detailed case example to demonstrate how the theory informed the treatment. Chapter 3 offers, instead of a single case, a series of organizing questions, frameworks and practical steps to help clinicians translate the theory into practice when doing short-term therapy. The summary of self psychology theory that opens Chapter 2 relies on Kohut's earliest formulations and excludes various subsequent developments in the theory and the concepts later used to discuss clinical phenomena. The emphasis was entirely on structure building via the internalization of selfobject functions as self functions, with optimal frustration described as a primary engine of growth. The findings of infant research, emphasizing self and mutual regulation, and the understanding from intersubjectivity theory that experience becomes organized and reorganized in specific relational contexts, were not yet available. Nevertheless, when the terms referenced in these chapters first appeared in Kohut's writings, they offered powerful new ways to understand and respond to our patients.

Chapter 4 continues the effort to extend and apply self psychological theory beyond the practice of psychoanalysis by using the concepts of self psychology to inform the process of clinical supervision and training. From this perspective, the supervisor forms an empathic alliance with the internal, subjective experience of the supervisee and focuses on the therapist-in-training's selfobject needs in order to facilitate the maintenance of their self-esteem and expansion of their cognitive understanding. Examples of these processes are illustrated by a series of vignettes, chosen from a variety of clinical settings and modalities of treatment.

Part Two of the book, consisting of Chapters 5, 6 and 7, involves interaction with the ideas of other self psychologists, writing in more contemporary terms. Responding to specific papers of theirs provided opportunities to offer more of my own ideas about particular topics not elaborated in the chapters in Part One.

Chapter 5 is a discussion of Dick Geist's paper on interpretation as a carrier of selfobject functions. This afforded me an opportunity to describe how the concept of interpretation has evolved, first after Freud and then after Kohut. I also review Kohut's theory of development, especially as elaborated by Marian Tolpin, and clarify how it dovetails with Geist's understanding of the mutative power of interpretation. Finally, I elaborate an idea that has become central to how I think about therapeutic action, i.e., the necessity of people shifting from a focus on external people and events to a focus on their internal experience. I describe the process by which we help them do so.

Chapter 6 is a discussion of George Hagman's work on self agency. In it I expand and elaborate upon our understanding of defense and the importance of forward edge interpretation in promoting a sense of personal agency. Hagman's clinical case material is used to further illustrate principles I outlined in the chapters on brief treatment. The chapter ends with comments on how the sense of agency can be both threatened and restored in the broader context of historical and political events.

Chapter 7 is a discussion of Magid, Shane and Fosshage's paper on relational self psychology. While the previous two chapters elaborated my ideas on interpretation, development, defense and the forward edge, in this discussion I add my thoughts about transference. I see this topic as central to the issue of asymmetry in the therapeutic relationship and believe that a focus on transference guides us to the steadfast focus on internal experience which I have been elaborating in previous chapters. These authors offer an extensive and helpful review of how our theory has evolved and changed over time. My discussion underscores the importance of also attending to the continuities in our theory.

Part Three, consisting of Chapters 8 and 9, pulls together many of the ideas threaded through the previous seven chapters. Chapter 8 describes the subtleties and complexities of empathic communication. It is a culmination of what I've gleaned from my years of practice, supervision and teaching regarding how to frame what we say to patients. Having seen that appreciating the importance of employing an empathic mode of observation and response does not necessarily mean that one knows how to do so effectively, in this chapter, especially, I aim to bridge this gap between theory and practice. I do so by offering a series of experience-near principles for enhancing the effectiveness of empathic communication, along with multiple representative examples of each. The chapter opens with a review of our contemporary understanding of the theoretical assumptions that underlie the focus on empathy, including those related to development, psychopathology and therapeutic action. Because the suggestions offered here emerged from the process of teaching, training and supervising mental health professionals in all disciplines, they are presented as a resource not only for clinicians, but also for teachers and supervisors.

Chapter 9 offers a retrospective summary of my journey toward becoming a self psychologist. I chose to end the book with this chapter, which originally was a Kohut Lecture I gave in Jerusalem in 2014, in hopes that it might both inspire and guide others in pursuing their own paths, as well as encouraging them to help others do so. Believing in the importance of both didactic and experiential learning, I trace formative experiences of mine in the realms of reading, meetings, mentors and personal therapy. I encourage and offer ways for readers to think about formative experiences in their own professional growth and underscore the importance of cross-fertilization across generations of younger and more seasoned clinicians.

I hope that this book will be helpful to the reader in achieving the goal of my title, translating theory into practice, and thereby unlocking the immense healing power of the ideas embodied in the psychology of the self.

References

Goldberg, A. (1985). The definition and role of interpretation. In A. Goldberg (Ed.), *Progress in self psychology* (Vol. 1, pp. 62–65). New York, NY: The Guilford Press.

Miller, J. (1985). How Kohut actually worked. In A. Goldberg (Ed.), *Progress in self psychology* (Vol. 1, pp. 13–30). New York, NY: The Guilford Press.

Strozier, C., Pinteris, K., Kelley, K., & Cher, D. (2022). *The new world of self: Heinz Kohut's transformation of psychoanalysis and psychotherapy*. New York, NY: Oxford University Press.

Tolpin, M. (2002). Doing psychoanalysis of normal development: Forward edge transferences. *Progress in Self Psychology*, *18*, 167–190.

Part One

Chapter 1

Self Psychology

Its Essence and Clinical Importance

At the annual meeting of the American Psychological Association in 2000, Theodore Millon organized a panel on the treatment of personality disorders from multiple theoretical perspectives, including family systems, cognitive behavioral and psychodynamic, among others. He invited me to address the topic from the viewpoint of self psychology. The talk was to be no longer than 10 minutes and would be addressed to an audience which would include many people who knew nothing at all about self psychology in particular or even psychoanalytic concepts in general. This required a statement that had to be comprehensive, but also extremely compact. Although it was never published, I include and begin with it in this volume as a kind of overview and summary of how one might describe the essence of self psychology as it was understood at the time and how it would inform the understanding and treatment of personality (or self) disorders.

This talk was presented on August 5, 2000, as "Self Psychology for the Personality Disorders" at the Annual Meeting of the American Psychological Association in Washington, DC.

Any theory of treatment for personality disorders rests on a set of assumptions about development and psychopathology. So let me start there. Self psychology evolved from the work of an analyst named Heinz Kohut, who was interested in narcissism. In the context of working with narcissistic personality disorders, Kohut (1971, 1984) identified a new form of transference, which came to be known as selfobject transference. He realized that these patients were looking for him to function as an extension of themselves, by offering experiences which would substitute for capacities which they were missing internally. What was being transferred onto the therapist, then, was the patient's thwarted developmental needs.

DOI: 10.4324/9781003491453-2

From this seminal observation, Kohut and others developed a theory which shifted the central focus in understanding motivation and development from the libidinal and aggressive drives to the maturation of a cohesive self. The self is an organization of experience, characterized by qualities of cohesiveness, vitality and a sense of continuity in time and space. It is developed and sustained by the empathic response of others (what self psychologists call an empathic selfobject milieu or matrix) who are required in order to meet basic and lifelong needs for vitalizing affective experiences. In other words, what drives us is a psychological need for the relational experiences that are necessary to sustain a cohesive sense of self.

When the child's need for empathic responsiveness is not adequately met by caregivers, development becomes derailed. This results in structural deficits and pathological defenses, the two problems which form the crux of personality (or self) disorders. Structural deficits are deficits in inner regulating capacities: self-soothing, self-righting and so forth. A self disorder is generally characterized by an inability to regulate affect and self-esteem. Pathological defenses are defenses erected to safeguard or restore the fragile self, to prevent further fragmentation and to ward off additional trauma. The unique pattern of defensive structures and structural deficits determines the specific nature of the personality disorder.

Behind the intrusive, chaotic and irritating behavior of the borderline patient is a desperate attempt to evoke urgently needed help in tension regulation. Behind the grandiose, entitled, demanding behavior of the narcissistic personality is an attempt to bolster very tenuous self-esteem.

Across the range of Axis II diagnoses, these problems leave patients with an inability to manage affect and meet needs in mature and age-appropriate forms. This creates a vicious cycle of unfulfilling relationships, failed goals and inadequate emotional nourishment.

Now let me turn to treatment. The goal of treatment is to strengthen the self, that is, to increase internal structure and functional capacities. Treatment involves the resumption of arrested development through the reactivation of thwarted developmental needs which are exposed and reworked in the transference. The process by which this occurs is through the use of an empathic mode of observation to understand the patient's subjective experience and through empathic interpretations to communicate that understanding to the patient.

It is a defining feature of self psychology to focus on inner life through empathic interpretations. We speak to subjective experience because that is the entry point to the patient's internal world. Empathic interpretations accept, understand and explain the meaning of the patient's experiences (A. Ornstein, 1986). They clarify and legitimize needs and affect. Empathic interpretations also facilitate the resolution of defenses. In this theory, symptoms, resistance and defense are all understood as adaptive responses to vulnerability and are interpreted as such. I'd like to offer three, brief examples.

In the first case, the patient flew into a rage and threatened to break off his engagement when his girlfriend announced that she would no longer continue her nightly ritual of putting his toothpaste on his toothbrush for him. Exploring and then reflecting his patient's subjective experience, the therapist said to him:

> It felt like such a betrayal when she suddenly said she wouldn't do it anymore ... you didn't know what you could count on from her. When she suddenly feels unreliable like that, it's like being right back in your family all over again and you feel so unsafe that you just have to get away from it.

As the therapist continued to explore and interpret the patient's experience along these lines, he was able to work through his feelings, accept the change in his girlfriend's behavior without residual anxiety or anger and stay in the relationship.

The next example is a brief excerpt from the second session of a psychotherapy case:

Pt: I don't understand why I am here with you, you're just going to send me home after we talk. Maybe I should leave now.

Th: It sounds like you're afraid that what we do here won't be enough. You're wondering if it's even worth it.

Pt: I have to be strong to take care of everyone else. No one would know what to do if *I* fell apart. Who would take care of me?

Th: You want to know that someone cares about you, but you're afraid no one would be there if *you* fell apart.

Pt: You don't care about me. You're only here because it's your job, picking people apart! You're supposed to open me up so you can see what's wrong with me, explain it to me, and then just when the going gets tough, you get going!

Th: So you expect that I'll open you up and then just leave you all alone to deal with what's wrong, right when you most need my help. From what you said earlier, this is something you have experienced before. You've gotten used to people getting inside you and then rejecting what they see. You're afraid that I will do the same thing, and you don't want to be hurt like that again.

At this point the patient began to cry. The therapist's empathic attunement enabled her to feel understood, in terms of both her wishes and her fears, i.e., the protective functions of her anger and defensiveness. Her affect changed markedly as she began to talk about earlier experiences of rejection, expressing painful feelings in a way she had previously been unable to do.

In my final example, the patient told his analyst at a Monday session that he had spent much of the previous weekend at public men's rooms, voyeuristically "peeking" at the other men. In the therapist's words:

He reported a sense of feeling bizarre. In a desolate voice, he reported having spent the times he was not in men's rooms painting empty chairs in his apartment. Suddenly he shouted, "I demand to know what you are thinking. You think I'm psychotic don't you?" [The therapist] replied, "I think you must have been very lonely." There was a pause, and then he burst out crying. When he was able to speak again, he said in a choked voice, "That was the first time anyone ever realized that." He paused again and added, "And I think that includes me."

(Goldberg, 1978, p. 271)

In describing the profound effect on the state of the self which this kind of empathic understanding has, P. Ornstein and Ornstein (1996) explained, "Feeling understood is the adult equivalent of being held, which on the level of self-experience results in firming up or consolidating the self" (p. 94). In other words, the therapist's empathic understanding and responsiveness create an atmosphere of safety and an increase in cohesion in the patient, which makes symptoms and defenses less necessary. The suspension of defense, in turn, makes it possible to access previously disavowed affects and needs. These can then be explored, integrated and transformed into more mature forms through the therapist's empathic responsiveness and interpretations. This process involves not only rational understanding, but also a new experience of self, other and the relationship between the two.

To summarize, empathic interpretations are used to communicate understanding, clarify experience, legitimize affect and needs, mitigate defensiveness and facilitate the reorganization of affective experience, all of which strengthen the self. In addition, for most patients the experience of being responded to in this way constitutes a new relational experience, which is in itself a potent aspect of the mutative process.

It has been said that if you pose a question to two Talmudic scholars, you can get five opinions. It's a bit like that within self psychology. So I've tried to limit myself to the most basic tenet of treatment upon which nearly all self psychologists would agree: Consistent use of an empathic mode of inquiry and interpretation, within the context of a therapeutic relationship, offers an exceptionally fruitful way to address the structural deficits and pathological defenses which form the core of the Axis II personality disorders.

References

Goldberg, A. (1978). *The psychology of the self: A casebook.* New York, NY: International Universities Press.

Kohut, H. (1971). *The analysis of the self.* New York, NY: International Universities Press.

Kohut, H. (1984). *How does analysis cure?* Chicago, IL: University of Chicago Press.

Ornstein, A. (1986). "Supportive" psychotherapy: A contemporary view. *Clinical Social Work Journal, 14,* 14–30.

Ornstein, P., & Ornstein, A. (1996). I. Some general principles of psychoanalytic psychotherapy: A selfpsychological perspective. In L. Lifson (Ed.), *Understanding therapeutic action: Psychodynamic concepts of cure* (pp. 87–101). Hillsdale, NJ: The Analytic Press.

Chapter 2

Application to Brief Psychotherapy

A Case Example

At the time this article was written, most of the published literature in self psychology illustrated the theory with clinical examples drawn from psychoanalysis or intensive psychoanalytic psychotherapy. This article, in contrast, sought to establish brief or time-limited psychotherapy as an appropriate domain for the application of self psychology. Primary emphasis was placed on assessing the state of the self and establishing a self-selfobject bond as the matrix for reinstating a previously arrested process of development, structure building and change.

Originally published in 1991, the article relies on Kohut's earliest formulations and excludes various subsequent developments in the theory of self psychology and in the concepts later used to discuss clinical phenomena. Kohut's use of the word structure was largely a remnant of the earlier language of the day in which psychoanalytic concepts were cast. Subsequent writers have spoken of the same phenomena more in terms of functional capacities and organizations of experience. People today rarely write in terms of "structure." Nor is transmuting internalization of the therapist's functions as self functions seen as the only way growth occurs. Instead, the findings of infant research have emphasized self and mutual regulation, while concepts from intersubjectivity theory have helped us understand how experience becomes organized and reorganized in specific relational contexts. Nevertheless, when the terms referenced in this article first appeared in his writings, these were tremendously important concepts in Kohut's theory. So, while the language has somewhat changed and we have expanded our understanding of development in new ways, I believe there are nevertheless a number of ideas in this chapter and the one that follows that remain quite true and useful. After a summary of basic concepts and review of relevant literature about brief treatment, the article

DOI: 10.4324/9781003491453-3

demonstrates how self psychological theory can be applied to brief treatment via a detailed case report.

This paper was published in 1991 as "The Application of Self Psychology to Brief Psychotherapy" in Psychoanalytic Psychology, *Volume 8.*

The theory of self psychology, as developed by Kohut (1966, 1971, 1977, 1984; Kohut & Wolf, 1978) and his followers (e.g., Goldberg, 1980a, 1983; Goldberg & Stepansky, 1984; Wolf, 1988), provides an integrated view of normal development, psychopathology and the treatment process. Although developed in the context of psychoanalysis and intensive, psychoanalytic psychotherapy, the conceptual framework offered by self psychology is applicable to a wide variety of settings in which clinicians practice. It particularly helps therapists to understand and intervene with a broad range of people who are vulnerable, either temporarily or chronically, to difficulties in maintaining self-esteem, regulating internal tension and accomplishing life goals.

My interest in writing this chapter emerged from my experience teaching and supervising people who were working in settings where frequency and duration of therapy were limited, either by clinic policy, third-party reimbursers or patient resources. Clinicians repeatedly expressed enthusiasm for the insights provided by the theory but felt confused about how to apply what they read to the settings in which they worked. As a way to bridge this gap, this chapter serves to illustrate how the theory of self psychology can be applied to time-limited psychotherapy. A brief summary of self psychological concepts is provided, followed by a review of the literature on self psychology and brief treatment, and then a detailed case example.

The Psychology of the Self—A Summary of Basic Concepts

Kohut defined the core of development as the maturation of a cohesive nuclear self. This self is imbued with basic strivings for power and success, basic idealized goals, and basic talents and skills (Kohut & Wolf, 1978).

The developing child has an exhibitionistic need for admiring, mirroring and confirming responses to his or her innate sense of vigor, greatness and perfection. Kohut (1971) referred to this dimension of the child's experience as the grandiose self. With appropriate mirroring, this early expansiveness matures into self-esteem, assertiveness, ambition, a healthy enjoyment of successes and a pleasure in the pursuit of interests and activities.

The child also has a need for closeness, contact, acceptance and support from an omnipotent, idealized source of calmness and strength. Kohut called this the idealized parent imago. When the child is permitted to merge with the idealized calmness and strength of parental selfobjects, these idealizing needs are transformed into ideals and values, idealized goals, and respect and admiration for others. Transformation of the idealized parent imago also leads to the capacity for self-soothing, self-comfort and self-regulation, particularly in regard to affects and tension states.

Finally, Kohut defined a basic need for twinship, the reassuring experience of essential alikeness, belonging and kinship with others. Appropriate human closeness and twinship (also called alter-ego) experiences lead to a capacity to utilize optimally one's talents and skills.

The emergence of the self requires the presence of others who provide selfobject experiences—experiences that will evoke and maintain the self's cohesion (Wolf, 1988). Selfobject refers to the internal, subjective experience of functions provided by others who are experienced as part of the self. Selfobject experiences are intrapsychic events which are not objectively observable. They are not object relations or interpersonal relations, although the latter may provide selfobject experiences (Wolf, 1988). The functions which selfobjects provide are mirroring, idealizing and alter-ego experiences.

Although these ideas were initially developed in the context of Kohut's work with narcissistically disordered patients, Kohut and others have expanded them into a general theory of human motivation and development. Self psychology holds that the guiding force in human development is the need for connections to sources of selfobject experiences throughout the entire course of life. The form that these experiences take changes as the relationship between self and selfobject matures (Wolf, 1980a), but the need does not go away. Kohut regarded this as a fundamental theoretical shift from the centrality of instinctual, biological drives to the motivational primacy of self experience, that is, the psychological need for a milieu of empathic selfobjects from birth until death (Kohut, 1984).

The adequacy of the early selfobject milieu in meeting the child's developmental needs is decisive in determining the fate of the emerging self. The nuclear self crystallizes in the matrix of a particular selfobject environment, through a process of psychological structure formation Kohut called transmuting internalization. In this process, minor, nontraumatic empathic failures on the part of essentially in-tune parental selfobjects lead to a gradual replacement of the selfobjects and their functions by a self and its functions. In other words, over the course of development, selfobject functions initially provided by others are internalized to become self functions, or inner psychic structure. Structure means having formerly external functions permanently in one's possession (Kohut, 1987). These functions include self-soothing, self-regulation and the maintenance of self-cohesion (M. Tolpin, 1971). With the acquisition of inner psychic structure, the self grows cohesive and firm.

When structuralization is incomplete, the loss of a selfobject is experienced as loss of part of the self and its needed functions. A variety of narcissistic injuries, separations or disruptions in relationships can precipitate this loss of requisite selfobject supplies. Such loss of needed selfobjects leads to fragmentation, enfeeblement, rage and various measures to keep the self together.

Psychopathology is caused by disturbances in the self-selfobject relations of childhood. If the environment fails to respond in phase-appropriate, non-traumatic ways to the needs of the child's developing self, the child's early grandiosity and wish to merge with an omnipotent selfobject cannot be transformed into reliable self-esteem, realistic ambitions and attainable ideals (Kohut, 1977). The underdeveloped self remains fragmented and empty, rather than cohesive, firm and vigorous. The problem is not one of conflict, as in classical libido theory, but of deficit: Normal development has been derailed and needs to be resumed. Treatment, then, involves strengthening or rehabilitating the self.

In a manner analogous to normal development, therapy aims to increase inner psychic structure, as selfobject functions initially performed by the therapist become self functions through the process of transmuting internalization. The strengthened self is better able to regulate tension and self-esteem, pursue nuclear ambitions and goals and enjoy empathic contact with mature selfobjects.

Kohut (1984) described the outcome of successful treatment in terms of both an increase in internal structure, reflected in greater firmness, cohesion and vigor of the patient's self, and an expansion of the patient's selfobject milieu, reflected in an increasing ability to identify, seek out and be sustained by appropriate selfobjects (both mirroring and idealizable) as currently available.

Therapeutic Processes

Kohut consistently emphasized the importance of looking at the patient's experience from within the patient's own perspective. The therapist gains access to this experience by the process of empathy. Kohut (1959, 1984) defined empathy as "vicarious introspection," a mode of observation which enables the therapist to grasp the affective state of the patient "while simultaneously retaining the stance of an objective observer" (1984, p. 175).

The therapist speaks to the patient's subjective experience and internal reality, conveying back whatever he or she understands the patient to be saying. In this process, the therapist focuses on experience and affect, helping the patient to organize and clarify the meaning of his or her experience, while underscoring the salient feelings in the patient's communications. In particular, the therapist articulates an empathic understanding and acceptance of the underlying needs, wishes, longings and motives expressed in the patient's behavior.

Affirming whatever expressions of self the patient offers enhances the patient's sense of the validity of his or her own experience. Faulty empathy in the past leads to a repudiation of needs that interferes with getting them met in the present. In contrast, when the therapist shares his or her sense of the legitimacy of the patient's needs, it makes it easier for the patient to integrate those needs and transform them into their mature counterparts (Kohut, 1984).

This empathic mode of listening and responding, which makes contact with the patient's inner experience and enlivens his or her communications (A. Ornstein, 1986), is the vehicle for engaging the patient in a therapeutic process and establishing a "therapeutic dialogue" (A. Ornstein & Ornstein, 1986). The therapist's clarifying comments about the subjective meaning of the events the patient reports help the patient learn to direct his or her attention inward and become introspective. The therapist's empathic responsiveness also creates an ambience and sense of safety that facilitate the patient's sharing and exploring aspects of himself or herself which initially were too threatening to allow into awareness. Once these previously repressed or disavowed dimensions of experience become part of the dialogue, the therapist is in a position to offer the patient empathic interpretations of them. Empathic interpretations accept, understand and explain the meaning of the patient's experiences (A. Ornstein, 1986). Such interpretations "bring relief by giving meaning to otherwise frightening and bewildering affects and thoughts" (P. Ornstein & Ornstein, 1977, p. 349).

Kohut (1959, 1984) defined empathy primarily as a mode of observation, a way of gathering the data needed to make empathic interpretations. It was the understanding and explanation of disruptions in the selfobject transference bond with the therapist that he saw as transforming a potential trauma into an experience of "optimal frustration" and leading to the accretion of psychic structure. However, Kohut (1973/1978) also described empathy as a "fundamental mode of human relatedness" (p. 704), a "powerful psychological bond" (p. 705) that serves as a nutriment to sustain human life as we know it. In his final article, he suggested that "empathy per se, the mere presence of empathy," might have a "therapeutic effect" (Kohut, 1982, p. 397).

Terman (1988, 1989) greatly elaborated this notion. He described how the empathic bond with the therapist and the patient's experience of being understood are intrinsic parts of structure formation and the curative process itself. Terman argued that being understood is growth producing in its own right, with the experience of a new relationship with the therapist enabling both the growth of new structure and the change of existing structure.

Stolorow (1986) similarly observed that:

> [The therapist's] consistent acceptance and empathic understanding of the patient's affective states and needs regularly come to be experienced by the patient as a facilitating medium reinstating developmental processes of self-articulation and self-demarcation that had been aborted and arrested during the formative years.
>
> (p. 397)

Stolorow's (1983) concept of "optimal empathy," Bacal's (1985) "optimal responsiveness" and P. Tolpin's (1988) "optimal affective engagement" all underscore the role of the therapist's responsiveness, rather than frustration, as the curative agent.

In his clarifications of the treatment process, Wolf (1988) described how for certain patients the therapeutic ambience itself is mutative:

> ... the accepting ambience of being in the presence of a respected person who is seriously, nonjudgmentally, and empathically interested in the patient's inner world may be the first such experience in their life. Treatment becomes the first occasion to be in a milieu that facilitates the healing of the self by allowing those aspects of the self which had been arrested in their development to resume developing.
>
> (p. 109)

This process occurs through the therapy relationship. Kohut (1984) described the reactivation of thwarted developmental needs as the essential driving force of the treatment process. The therapist, functioning as a new selfobject and responding to the patient's emerging transference needs, reactivates development at the point at which earlier attempts to secure appropriate response from selfobjects failed (Elson, 1986). The patient's selfobject demands are viewed as legitimate expressions of his or her wish for the therapist to provide missing intrapsychic functions. In response to the patient's search for responses to these legitimate needs for structure building, the therapist performs selfobject functions that can be transmuted into self functions, or inner psychic structure.

When the problem that brings the patient to treatment reflects a loss of previously established cohesion or vigor due to narcissistic injury or other disruptions in needed selfobject supplies, the therapist similarly responds to the patient's selfobject needs in ways which allow the patient to restore his or her self to the previous level of functioning.

It is not that the therapist actively tries to put himself or herself in the role of selfobject, but rather that the patient's needs and the spontaneous transference of those needs put the therapist in this role (M. Tolpin, 1983). When the therapist is then optimally responsive to these needs, which arise out of deficits in prior selfobject relationships, a corrective or therapeutic selfobject experience occurs (Bacal, 1990).

Brief Treatment and Self Psychology

The rather extensive literature on short-term, dynamic psychotherapy (for excellent summaries, see Budman, 1981; Donovan, 1987) contains very few articles written explicitly from a self psychological perspective. Case material published by Kohut and his followers (e.g., Goldberg, 1978), on the other hand, primarily reports on psychoanalysis or long-term psychoanalytic psychotherapy, the clinical data from which the theory of self psychology was derived.

There are some exceptions. Books by Basch (1980, 1988), Kohut (1987) and Elson (1986), though not about short-term psychotherapy *per se*, do include a number of brief treatment cases which were informed by the authors' self psychological perspective. Although he didn't write on the topic extensively, Kohut saw his ideas as very relevant for brief treatment.

Speaking to workers in a university mental health clinic, Kohut (1987) encouraged them not to underestimate the importance of this modality. He felt that a little bit of help, emanating from the borrowed strength of the therapist's support, could accomplish a great deal.

Goldberg (1973) offered perhaps the earliest explicit attempt to apply the evolving insights of self psychology to short-term psychotherapy. Discussing the psychotherapeutic treatment of narcissistic injuries, he described a need for the patient to be able to use the therapist as a source of mirroring, twinship or idealizing selfobject functions in order to restore self-esteem. It was specifically in the understanding and interpretation of the patient's frustrated selfobject longings that repair of the injured self was seen to occur. Goldberg (1980b) later elaborated a concept of psychotherapy, as distinct from psychoanalysis, which emphasized the repair of the self as its defining feature.

Lazarus (1980) also applied self psychology to brief treatment. Like Goldberg, he conceptualized the goal of brief therapy with narcissistic disturbances as one of reestablishing the patient's feelings of self-esteem and self-cohesion by allowing the patient to use the therapist as a selfobject. He saw the outcome of brief therapy as limited, in most cases, to reinstatement of the patient's pre-morbid level of functioning and self-esteem. He believed that in some cases, however, the patient might begin to internalize the therapist's functions, leading to an accretion of internal psychic structure and promoting further insight and working through of narcissistic problems after termination.

In a later article, Lazarus (1988) described the use of self psychological principles to conduct brief psychotherapy with elderly patients whose entry into treatment was similarly precipitated by a narcissistic injury or other selfobject loss. Lazarus again described how the relationship with the empathic therapist may serve as a bridge to restore self-esteem and help the patient reestablish a supportive selfobject milieu outside of the treatment context.

The most detailed case report of an effort to bring self psychology and brief treatment together is provided by Chernus's (1983) description of the use of focal psychotherapy to treat a structural defect in the self.[1] Chernus defined focal psychotherapy as a specific variety of brief psychotherapy in which therapist and patient explore and work through a focal conflict precipitated by a recent event that has overwhelmed the patient's characterological defense mechanisms.[2]

In conducting focal psychotherapy with a patient whose primary problem was conceptualized as a structural deficit in the self, Chernus expanded the terrain described by others. In the case she reported, the primary therapeutic goals were structure building and internalization of the therapist's selfobject functions. In contrast, other reports of focal psychotherapy had emphasized conflict resolution or defense analysis, whereas other reports of brief, self psychological treatment had emphasized repair of the self and return to pre-morbid levels of functioning.

Chernus also suggested that the briefer the treatment, the more likely it was that the weight of the working-through process would occur in the context of the patient's external relationships and experiences, rather than in the transference to the therapist. The therapeutic relationship was seen as important for what it exposed of these other experiences. P. Ornstein and Ornstein (1972) similarly found that working through occurred in meaningful ways outside of the therapeutic relationship.

In any kind of brief or time-limited treatment, the therapist must decide where to put his or her therapeutic energy, given limited resources. All forms of brief therapy address the issue of focus in one way or another. From a self psychological perspective, the choice is clear: The focus must be on the state of the patient's self and on the relationship between the patient and therapist as a new self-selfobject unit. This means that the therapist: (a) attends specifically to ways in which the self is vulnerable, injured or arrested; (b) understands symptomatic expressions both outside and within the therapy relationship as manifestations of these deficits; and (c) enables the patient to establish the selfobject matrix required to facilitate the self's repair and growth. This is the guiding beacon for all of the therapist's activities.

A. Ornstein (1986) suggested that concern with the state of the self should be the primary focus in the treatment of all patients, regardless of the nature of the pathology or form of the treatment. She reported that even in once-weekly therapy, feeling understood can lead to an increase in self-cohesion which allows an exploration of affects, wishes, fears and fantasies that had previously been repressed or disavowed because of their threat to self-cohesion. The emergence of these previously unavailable aspects of the patient's experience into awareness provides an opportunity to understand their meaning and, in so doing, to use the therapy relationship to strengthen the self.

Elson (1986) reached a similar conclusion:

> Self psychology clarifies the universal striving to secure a response to
> one's potential for individuality and significance. In even the most seri-
> ously deprived individual, underneath abrasive and cynical behavior, a
> vestige of the need to be confirmed remains alive to be rekindled. The
> very presence of the [therapist] may quicken this need. Many methods and
> approaches have been devised for responding to and controlling the rela-
> tionship which ensues, but, regardless of method, how one orders what
> one sees and experiences, how one uses oneself on behalf of the individ-
> ual, becomes more vivid through an explanatory system of human behav-
> ior that places the self of the individual at the center of one's observations
> and views the new self/selfobject unit as the medium for treatment.
>
> (p. 136)

The principles just described are illustrated in the following case report.
The patient was seen in a community mental health center where treatment is generally limited to 20 sessions. Guided by a self psychological formulation of the patient's difficulties and the treatment process,
the therapist's primary focus was on the self experience of the patient
and the formation of a self-selfobject bond as a matrix for change.
An empathic-introspective mode was used to engage the patient and
develop the treatment process. Selected segments of the treatment are
presented in detail and in the patient's own words, in order to provide
the reader with an experience of the unfolding therapeutic and developmental process.

Case Example: Jim[3]

Jim, an 18-year-old college freshman, was brought to the hospital emergency room after taking an overdose of medications. Although he mentioned an argument with his girlfriend, Carol, as a precipitant for this action,
he was unable to explain what had caused him to impulsively swallow all
the pills in the family medicine chest. His mother, who accompanied him
to the hospital, said she'd had no idea that her son was having problems
and was equally baffled by his action. Jim agreed to see a therapist at the
hospital's outpatient mental health center, where he was assigned to a psychology intern and seen for the first session two days later. His original

20-session contract was extended briefly, and he was seen for a total of 25 weekly visits.

In the first few sessions, Jim displayed little self-awareness and extremely restricted affect. He was formal, polite and guarded, making little eye contact and no spontaneous comments. He was unable to associate to open-ended questions and responded to direct questions with articulate but very brief answers. History was reported with no show of emotion. The therapist worried about how she would be able to use an empathic mode to engage this young man, who seemed so unable to articulate his inner experience.

Jim had no idea why he took all the pills following his argument with Carol. After doing so, it occurred to him that "I might die," which was "scary," and he forced himself to vomit. When he then told his mother he thought he should go to the hospital, she and his stepfather drove him there in total silence, asking no questions. Jim reported that he has little communication with his mother and stepfather, but that their relationship has "no problems." He agreed to a 20-session therapy contract, saying "I never want anything like this [overdose] to happen again." The goals he identified for treatment were to understand why he swallowed the pills and to be able to talk with the significant people in his life about the overdose.

Jim lives with his mother, stepfather and brother, Al, who is a year younger and his only sibling. His parents divorced when he was 9 and his father moved to another part of the country, visiting his sons only once or twice a year after that. Jim was unable to express any feelings about this situation. After the divorce, Jim's family moved to his maternal grandmother's home. He became very attached to this grandmother, who died suddenly of a stroke when he was 13. When Jim was 17, his mother got remarried to a man whom Jim described as "a nice guy, he used to be my coach." Jim also mentioned his cousin, Ted, as being his "best friend." Carol had been Jim's girlfriend for 10 months, his first serious romantic relationship. He mentioned that they have frequent arguments but was unable to describe one, saying that he can't remember them afterwards.

In talking about his college courses, Jim expressed uncertainty about what he wanted to study or do with his life. He had hoped to go away to a state college where he had been accepted, but switched at the last minute to a local community college when his parents announced, just two weeks before he was to leave, that they couldn't afford the state school because they were still paying his brother's parochial school tuition. Jim spoke matter-of-factly about this change in plans. When asked how he felt about it, he replied, "It's no big deal."

As Jim responded to her initial inquiries, the therapist increasingly developed a picture of a young man with significant problems in recognizing and managing his affective experience. His entry into treatment was precipitated by a suicidal gesture triggered by feelings he was so out of touch with that he described it almost as a dissociative event. He had no idea where it came from, but something broke through, frightened him and got his attention—he experienced a fear that he might die. Jim's difficulty in affect regulation became an important focus of the therapist's attention.

In these early sessions, the therapist tried to latch onto whatever glimpses of self-expression Jim offered, reflecting them back to him as a way to direct his attention inward and invite him to say more. He began describing how he wished he could figure out how to tell his girlfriend what his needs are without causing fights. Freedom to "go out with the guys" was a particular wish of his. He expressed frustration over his perceived choices either to express his desires and make her angry, to do what she wants and miss out on other things he enjoys, or to do what he wants without telling her and risk her getting "even madder" if she finds out.

Although Jim could describe Carol's anger, he said that he himself should not get mad, because that would cause a "really big fight." The therapist commented that anger seemed to feel kind of dangerous to him, and Jim agreed. By commenting on his sense of danger, the therapist tried not only to help Jim identify his feelings, but also to offer an empathic appreciation of the protective functions that his defenses against affective awareness and expression were serving.

As the therapist helped Jim explore these issues, eye contact increased and their verbal interactions became more comfortable. Jim experimented briefly with dating a girl in one of his classes, which led to Carol's giving him back his class ring. "It wasn't so much that she was mad at me; it was more that her feelings were hurt and she was confused." Jim broke off the new relationship and returned to Carol, because he realized "we had more in common." Noting the gains in awareness reflected in these statements, the therapist commented that Jim seemed to have learned some important things about both himself and Carol through experimenting with another relationship.

The therapist's empathy both modeled and encouraged introspection, as Jim learned to take her accepting attitude toward himself. His beginning identification with and internalization of the therapist's functions and attitude about exploring feelings became even more evident when Jim proudly announced that, since getting back together with Carol, he had "played psychiatrist" for her. He said this had led her to talk more openly than ever before and that they had reached "new levels of intimacy" in their communication. Very pleased with this new development, Jim announced, "Maybe I'll be a psychiatrist like you!" The opportunity to merge with his therapist's calm and guiding understanding of his inner life had clearly intensified Jim's idealization of her, as well as allowed him to begin transmuting some of her functions as he tried them out for himself.

Jim arrived at the seventh session with his hand in a cast. He explained that he and Carol had started arguing on the phone and in frustration he had hit the floor, cracking a bone in his hand. Because this time he had not swallowed pills, he said he felt he was making progress, but slowly. The therapist affirmed this, commenting that both times he had done something to harm himself physically before seeming to think about it. But a cracked bone isn't life threatening, so this felt less scary to him. Jim agreed.

Jim also reported that he had been spending more time with his cousin, Ted, rather than being with Carol all the time, and it felt like a better balance. Affirming Jim's initiative in trying to meet his own needs, the therapist observed that he had previously mentioned his wish for more freedom to do things separately from Carol, and he seemed to be figuring out how to arrange it.

Jim went on to describe how he had decided to try cooking dinner for Carol one night. He enjoyed surprising and pleasing her, and found it fun to try something new.

In the eighth session, Jim reported that people had been commenting that he talks more lately, which both surprised and pleased him. He attributed the change to "learning to talk here." He had told only Carol that he "sees a shrink," but he was considering telling Ted as well. Again noting his gains in self-expression, the therapist commented, "So you're talking more frequently, and now you're thinking about talking more intimately." Jim smiled and nodded.

As his self continued to grow more cohesive through his stabilizing tie with the selfobject therapist, Jim was able to begin to experience and integrate affects that he previously had needed to disavow. He reported, in the next session, that he had been "much more aware of emotional feelings." During the past week he had been in touch with painful feelings of loss about his grandmother's death and his father's "desertion" of him after the divorce. He added that during the week he had cried about these losses "for the first time ever." He said, "I thought I'd handled things so well during the divorce and at my grandmother's funeral because I never cried." The therapist listened quietly while Jim shared these painful memories. She then commented on how hard it must have been for Jim to have such sad feelings bottled up for so many years, how lonely and shut off he must have felt. Upon hearing this, Jim's body relaxed completely. He appeared visibly relieved in response to finally having someone who could understand, share in and absorb these feelings.

When a friend of Jim's was hospitalized psychiatrically, Jim remembered his own "close call," as he, too, had come to the hospital after suicidal behavior. But he observed that his friend was still unable to understand or talk about what was wrong. In contrast, Jim thought that in his own therapy he was making progress in both his self-understanding and self-expression.

He described "little fights" with Carol lately "but no big ones." He was enjoying a balance of activities with Carol, Ted, Al and "guys." With the cast off his hand, he joined a recreational basketball league, which he described as a lot of fun. He also found a summer job and was looking forward to an impending visit from his father for his brother's high school graduation.

In anticipating the start of his new job as an office clerk, Jim became nauseous and anxious, but was fine after he actually started. He also reported having a "fight" with Carol without "losing my cool." Jim was proud of his impulse control and mastery. At Carol's request, he also reduced his smoking. He was pleased that he had been able to do so and that she cared enough about him to be interested in his health.

Although Jim had still not been able to describe in any detail the argument that led to his suicidal behavior, it became possible, in the 14th session, to explore some of its deeper roots.

Discussing his feelings related to his father's recent visit, Jim reported that he had made the "interesting" discovery that his father's birthday coincided with the date of his suicidal gesture. He expressed his sense of hurt and anger over the fact that his father had come for his brother's graduation this year but had skipped Jim's graduation last year. He also was able to articulate his feelings of desertion and abandonment when his father moved away after the divorce nine years earlier. These associations allowed the therapist to discuss with Jim the possibility that on the night of his overdose, his argument with Carol had likewise triggered feelings of anger, desertion and abandonment, reverberating with similar feelings that had been bottled up since his father left.

Following this session, Jim reported having made another "discovery" over the weekend which so excited him that he had considered trying to reach his therapist to share it. But because they met on Mondays, he had decided he could wait one more day. Increasingly cognizant of his own needs for mirroring, affirmation and support, Jim said he realized that if someone close to him, like his mother or girlfriend, tells him that he will never be able to do something, then it becomes a self-fulfilling prophecy. But if the other person expresses confidence that he can accomplish something, then he is almost certain to be successful at it. He offered his efforts to stop smoking as an example.

Jim was able to explain this to Carol and that "felt great inside." The therapist listened attentively while Jim explained his new insights to her. She then reflected back what he'd said, while Jim nodded enthusiastically and frequently exclaimed, "Yeah!" Mirroring his enthusiasm, the therapist commented that he really was getting high on understanding himself lately. Jim laughed and said again that it felt pretty exciting.

Jim clearly was feeling a great sense of efficacy at this point. Joining with his therapist in this task of understanding his experience, he was able to transmute her selfobject functions into capacities of his own. He enjoyed the sense of control and mastery he felt as his self continued to grow in cohesion. With the developmental process reinstated, he also showed continued growth and pleasure in self-expression.

The therapist reminded Jim that they were in their 15th session and had five sessions left. Jim immediately said that he wanted five or ten extra sessions, "because I think this is good for me."

The following week Jim announced that he wanted Carol to meet his therapist and sit in on one of their sessions. He explained that after he stopped seeing the therapist he hoped to be able to talk to Carol about things that are on his mind. So he wanted her to "see how this works." Jim was trying to prepare the ground for an expansion of his selfobject milieu in which Carol would be able to provide some of the sustaining functions for which he had come to rely upon the therapist. After exploring the meaning of his request further, the therapist told Jim that he was welcome to bring Carol to a session if he and she both so desired. Jim also reiterated his request for an extension of therapy. He decided to ask for five extra sessions, because "I don't feel ready to end in just one month, but I don't want to go on forever either." The therapist subsequently obtained approval for this request.

Jim brought Carol to the next session. He responded to her visible nervousness by reassuring her that the therapist was "not going to analyze" her. Carol then sat quietly through the session as Jim, true to his word, showed her how it worked. He talked about his job experiences and his mother's pressure on him to take a math placement test. He explained his need to make choices for himself rather than be forced into doing things according to someone else's arbitrary schedule. The therapist helped him relate these feelings to her reminder of the impending termination and the clinic's "arbitrary schedule" of 20 sessions, which he had requested be changed to a number that felt more comfortable to him.

In the 19th session, the depth of Jim's deficits in affect and tension regulation were dramatically revealed, as the safety of his relationship with the therapist allowed him to share material he was previously "too embarrassed" to discuss. He described a variety of efforts to soothe himself at bedtime, which he called "bad habits." He said he had slept with a baby blanket until his mother took it away from him and burned it when he was 12. "I was pretty mad at her about that. I guess I still am!" He added that he had always sucked his thumb to go to sleep. "My mother hated that too. She used to put stuff on my thumb that would burn my tongue or make me gag. She doesn't know I still do it." More recently, Jim had smoked pot some nights if he felt "too uptight to sleep." His mother did not know about this, but Carol did and she strongly disapproved.

Jim's difficulty with the development of internal, self-soothing mechanisms contributed to his problem regulating his impulses and feelings, as manifested in his overdose, broken hand and initial isolation of affect. The therapist understood his "bad habits" as reflections of self deficits in these areas.

Jim's report of his mother's behavior suggested a longstanding lack of attunement to his needs, which the therapist's responses belatedly legitimized. She commented that it must seem to him as if the women closest to him could not recognize or would not accept that he has emotional needs. He replied that when he can hold Carol he relaxes completely and does not need any of the other devices. The therapist observed that what Jim really seemed to need when he's anxious is the natural comfort of human closeness with someone he loves. When it is there, he does not need the so-called "bad habits," which are all substitute ways of trying to provide something that is missing.

At the 20th session, Jim brought Carol in again. This time she participated actively. They wanted to discuss a topic they had been "fighting about" and to get the therapist's help. After listening for a while, the therapist concluded that they had in fact negotiated the issue very well and reached a mutual agreement. She shared this perception and supported their efforts to try to look at controversies from each other's perspective. They appeared very gratified by this validation of their new skills and left smiling, hand-in-hand.

When Jim returned, he reported more vignettes of negotiating issues with Carol and reconciling differences. He appeared relaxed and self-confident. He talked about his summer job and how he had been picturing himself in the various positions that existed in the large company where he worked. He thought he might be comfortable in the accounting department; he liked what he observed there and also what the men said about their jobs. He thought he would register for an accounting and business curriculum in the fall, "to try it on for size." Again the therapist listened attentively, occasionally making comments such as "you've got some real career possibilities in mind now." With his own ambition freed up, Jim was now able to explore vocational interests.

Jim also talked about wanting to learn to play the guitar. He shared fantasies about forming a rock band with his cousin, Ted, as another career possibility. Expounding on the possibilities, he speculated expansively and joyfully about great rock concerts they might perform. He then grinned and said even though this would probably never happen, they could have a lot of fun anyway. The therapist reflected back that he seemed to be having fun just thinking about it. It was to the now liberated, natural expansiveness of the child in Jim, long subdued by developmental arrest, that the therapist provided belated affirmation in making this comment. By accepting his dreams and joyfully sharing in Jim's grandiose-exhibitionistic fantasies, the therapist facilitated a process by which they could be transformed into realistic ambitions.

In the 23rd session, Jim brought a cassette of music he listened to every time he came to therapy: Led Zeppelin. He reported feeling sad that they would be ending in two sessions, which seemed "okay, but soon." He had felt like calling the therapist the night before but thought he should not. Instead he listened to the tape and decided to bring it to her. The tape clearly had taken on valence as a transitional object (Winnicott, 1951/1958; see also M. Tolpin, 1971), associated with the selfobject therapist and her soothing functions. In listening to it, Jim sought not only to soothe himself in the therapist's absence, but also to gain mastery over the more permanent separation from her which was rapidly approaching. The therapist empathized with his struggle to deal with all the feelings he had about their termination.

Jim also reported having had an argument on the phone with Carol and hitting the wall with the same hand in which he had previously cracked a bone. But this time he had hit with the fleshy side of his hand, so he broke some blood vessels but no bones. The therapist commented on this tangible increase in tension regulation and impulse control. She noted that Jim's impulsive actions had gotten much less damaging: A bruise heals faster than a bone, and neither is nearly as dangerous as a medication overdose. Jim replied that he felt sure he would never overdose again.

Although it is not clear that Jim had achieved total insight into the meaning of his overdose, he had achieved an important increase in self cohesion which allowed him to get in touch with and manage the affects associated with the loss of his father and his arguments with Carol. It was these affects, walled off (disavowed), which led to his dangerously destructive behavior. His vastly improved ability to know about and handle such feelings, along with his increased capacity for self-righting and self-soothing (M. Tolpin, 1983), gave credence to his conviction that he would not overdose again. He now had other alternatives.

Jim added that he had gotten a new dog during the week, only the second one he had ever owned, and said, "She's great!" His first dog had been put to sleep 10 years earlier. The therapist commented that the dog's death was yet another loss, but that now Jim felt he could make an attachment to this new pet, just as he was finding he could make attachments to new people in his life.

In the second to last session, Jim continued to manifest a freeing up and maturation in the grandiose pole of his self. He described how he was beginning to enjoy and look forward to his life; he wanted to plan a career and set goals for himself. He spoke of a wish "to put my mark on the world, maybe get my name in a book." He reported that such ambitions were new feelings, because he "never really cared what happened before."

His upcoming birthday, along with his termination from therapy, was leading Jim to "take inventory" of the year's progress. After doing research to choose an instrument and instructor, he told his mother he wanted a guitar for his birthday.

Jim said he wanted the therapist to keep the music tape he had given her, to listen to it and to think of him. He also requested that she give him something of hers, perhaps an old mug. She agreed to do so. This requested exchange of possessions reflected Jim's efforts to maintain his connection with the therapist in the face of their impending separation. During most of the session, the therapist listened quietly, while reflecting internally on just how much he had developed in the previous six months. As Jim was leaving, he wiped a few tears from his eyes.

In the final session, Jim spoke of having talked to Carol about his father's leaving and about his grandmother's death. He was able to express his feelings and cry with her, which "felt great" afterward. The therapist commented on how Jim seemed to have begun the process which he had hoped would happen after his therapy ended: to be able to talk to Carol the way he had talked to the therapist. He said that he and Carol had also discussed the possibility of eventual marriage and children.

After reviewing together Jim's progress during the course of therapy, Jim told the therapist that he felt "kind of good" about finishing treatment, because it's sort of like a graduation, but he also felt "kind of bad" because he would miss their sessions together. These comments reflected a vast increase in Jim's self-delineation regarding feelings. The nuances of emotion he was able to be aware of and verbalize about the termination stand in stark contrast to his behavior at the outset of treatment.

The therapist gave him an old mug, as he had requested and, being a guitarist herself, also offered him two of her guitar picks. Reflecting his continued attachment to and idealization of the therapist, Jim immediately said the picks would always be his favorites. Although he was surprised to learn that his therapist played the guitar, he was clearly delighted with these transitional selfobject gifts. He thanked the therapist for her help and said he might like to check in some time. She replied that she would be happy to hear from him and would be thinking about him in any case.

Approximately a year later, when the therapist called Jim to seek permission to publish a summary of his therapy, he reported that he was continuing in an accounting program, had obtained a guitar and was excited about having earned enough money through a part-time job to buy a used car. He was no longer seeing Carol, which he expressed some sadness about. Overall, he said he was doing fine.

Discussion

Over the course of treatment, Jim displayed maturation in nearly all sectors of his self experience: the development of ambition, use of talents and skills, and capacity for affect and tension regulation. This maturation is reflected in his pursuit of new activities, interests and goals and in his ability to put feelings into words, expressing upset verbally rather than in self-destructive behavior.

Socarides and Stolorow (1984–1985) suggested that selfobject functions pertain fundamentally to the integration of affect and that the central curative element in therapy is the role of the selfobject transference bond in the "articulation, integration and developmental transformation of the patient's affectivity" (p. 112). Certainly the changes in Jim's affective functioning over the course of treatment support this focus.

Miller (1991) also suggested that the central underlying process in psychotherapy is the formation of a selfobject bond with the therapist, which strengthens the patient's self functioning and increases structure. He went even further, suggesting that the formation, maintenance and internalization of this bond is the reason all treatments that work do so, regardless of the theoretical model espoused.

It is very clear in Jim's case that the internalization of the bond was incomplete at the time of termination. His use of the transitional objects exchanged with the therapist illustrates the sort of "psychic way station" which M. Tolpin (1971, p. 327) described as an intermediate step in the internalization of self-soothing functions.

The total silence in which Jim's family traveled to the hospital following his overdose speaks volumes about the emotional climate in his home: Feelings could not be discussed. His mother's response to his prolonged use of his baby blanket and thumb is another example of the absence of the selfobject support needed to integrate emotions and develop self-soothing capacities successfully. The therapist's response to these issues provided the kind of "corrective emotional dialogue" (M. Tolpin, 1983) that allowed Jim to resume a process of structure building in these areas.

Terminating with such important developments still in progress is neither unusual nor necessarily problematic in the context of brief psychotherapy, where the goal is often less to get something finished than to get something started. Whether what is started is a process of understanding, of stabilization or of change, the primary goal is a strengthening of the self, through which the patient may find new internal and external resources with which to go forward in dealing with life's challenges.

Therapists working under the constriction of time-limited sessions often feel pressured to curb what they see as unrealistic demands or self-destructive behavior in order to facilitate a more rapid adaptation by the patient to his or her life situation. In my experience, this inevitably leads to defensiveness and resistance, rather than more rapid progress.

It is, in fact, by consistently understanding, accepting and explaining the meaning of the patient's demands that the therapist is more rapidly able to help the patient change. I agree strongly with Goldberg (1973) that it is particularly the patient's frustrated selfobject longings that need to be acknowledged and affirmed as legitimate. It is when patients feel fully understood and accepted *vis-à-vis* their own experience as lived that they can begin to explore possibilities beyond their current awareness.

Jim's therapist put major emphasis on helping him appreciate the legitimacy of his needs and feelings. Armed with this newfound awareness, understanding and acceptance of his own experience, Jim was able to assert himself more actively in expanding his selfobject milieu. Nowhere was this more apparent than in the growth toward mature "empathic resonance" (Kohut, 1984, p. 66) evidenced in his relationship with Carol.

It is worth nothing that Jim's therapist was an intern, relatively new to practicing psychotherapy in general and totally new to self psychology in particular. Trainees in a time-limited setting are particularly vulnerable to feeling they have to do more if the patient is to improve in the allotted time. What was critical to Jim's therapist's ability to work so successfully with him was her capacity to be sensitively attuned to his needs and her having a theoretical perspective that allowed her to appreciate the meaning of those needs as they unfolded in the treatment. In making herself available to Jim as a new selfobject through whom the thrust to continue development could be resumed, she offered guiding strength and calmness, affective participation and needed affirmation of his experience. Once one can appreciate the therapeutic potency of such interventions, there is much less temptation to depart from the central focus of strengthening the self.

When the state of the self is the organizing focus of the therapist's interventions, certain technical decisions can also be made more easily and naturally. Certainly more traditional norms of technique might have militated against Jim's girlfriend coming in and out of his therapy as she did, or the therapist "gratifying" his request by actually giving him a mug of hers, let alone an additional gift of her own choosing. Yet her decisions about these events essentially followed her central goal: To provide the optimally responsive (Bacal, 1985, 1990; Bacal & Newman, 1990) selfobject availability that would foster the patient's growth. Allowing Jim to bring his girlfriend to sessions after the subject of termination had been raised facilitated his avowed desire to shift his needs from the therapist to this more ongoing relationship in his life. In providing the mug, the therapist appreciated Jim's struggle to internalize their bond and the functions it provided. She recognized that he felt a need for assistance from her in the form of a tangible transitional object as a way station in the process. In other words, what she "gratified" was his wish to be understood in the present, particularly in relation to his difficulty ending a relationship which had come to be so important to his renewed process of structure building. Similarly, her addition of the guitar picks was a way of both affirming his newly expressed interest in learning to play the guitar and letting him know that they had something in common. Idealizing, mirroring and twinship functions were all evident in the therapist's offering of these parting "gifts."

An alternative, of course, would have been to recognize and affirm verbally the needs expressed in Jim's request. It is not that the tangible exchange of possessions *per se* is advocated here, but rather that such interactions should be understood in the context of the patient's self experience. The real gift, ultimately, is the acquisition of those self functions which would enable Jim to maintain his own sense of vitality and cohesion. It is a focus on the strengths, vulnerabilities, longings and needs of the self which puts therapists in the best position to deal with these practical issues of technique and intervention.

Virtually any of the techniques described in other forms of psychotherapy might potentially be relevant and helpful in this kind of treatment. But techniques can never substitute for theory. In a sense, the key intervention lies in the therapist's own mindset. The therapist must have an organizing theoretical perspective for understanding what the patient presents and what the patient needs in order to change.

The mindset proposed here is the one that was described earlier: a focus on the self experience of the patient and on the relationship between the patient and therapist as a new self-selfobject unit. The selfobject dimension of the patient's experience, in particular, must be kept in sharp relief. Initially, this focus involves looking at the meaning of precipitating events in terms of their impact on the self's vitality and cohesion. The stresses people report as causing them to seek treatment often involve the loss of important selfobject functions, whether supplied directly by a relationship or by more symbolic activities and pursuits such as work and other interests. Similarly, symptoms should be examined for ways in which they express either a loss of the self's cohesion and vitality or attempts to soothe and restore the weakened self.

It is especially in the patient's behavior toward the therapist that the therapist must recognize what needs of the self are being expressed and affirm their legitimacy. This is of particular importance in brief psychotherapy, because misperceptions in this area lead to stalemates or entrenchments which may not be resolved in the limited number of sessions available.

The patient who wants to "chat," for example, may not be resisting other topics but rather searching for some kind of emotional participation with the therapist. The patient who clamors for advice and direction may be hoping the therapist will provide the idealizing functions of organizing and making sense out of his or her experience. The patient who provides detailed descriptions of his or her activities and accomplishments may be seeking mirroring and affirmation. On the other hand, patients who engage in hostile, provocative behavior toward the therapist may be desperately trying to shield themselves from the fear that their vulnerable self will again be traumatized by being rejected or misunderstood. Whatever the need, recognizing and affirming its legitimacy strengthens the self. Failure to do so threatens the self and may lead to an intensification of symptoms. The resulting impasse may also create negative countertransference feelings and a lowering of professional self-esteem in the therapist, who feels helpless, puzzled and frustrated by his or her inability to help the patient.

It is here especially that the theory is so important and so helpful. The more we understand our patients' symptomatic behavior as expressions of legitimate needs, or desperate attempts to hold together a crumbling self, the less likely we are to label them as resisting, acting out or being manipulative. When we see ourselves as being used by the patient in a necessary and appropriate way for missing functions and structure, we don't feel exploited, manipulated or helpless; we feel needed and useful. The stalemates and resulting frustration that therapists (especially beginning ones) feel toward their patients often stem from this failure to appreciate accurately the patient's needs and motives. Understanding phenomena from the point of view of the patient's subjective experience enables the therapist to offer the selfobject responsiveness the patient is desperately seeking. This, in turn, restores cohesion and allows symptoms to abate.

This is a familiar process, described by all writers in self psychology, in the context of healing empathic ruptures. What I think is different in brief treatment is the need for the therapist to continually articulate his or her understanding of the patient's experience and frustrated selfobject longings in a very explicit, active way. This could, of course, be helpful in any treatment, but it becomes imperative when the time available for therapy is limited.

The literature on self psychology and brief psychotherapy is so scant that little has been established regarding who might or might not benefit from this form of treatment. Clearly a minimum requirement is that a certain degree of cohesion has already been established. For people with very severe and long-standing deficits in internal self-regulating structure, a much more protracted period of therapeutic engagement is needed in order to realize significant improvement. Nor can this form of treatment necessarily clarify the deepest roots of the patient's pathology. P. Tolpin suggested that not only duration but also frequency of sessions is critical in reaching the "depths of the personality" (1991, p. 63) and the "primary injury of the core self" (1985, p. 86). The brief psychotherapy described here does not attempt to address these issues. Rather, the emphasis is on repair of the self and the freeing up of an arrested developmental process.

We can speculate that in Jim's case the marked improvement was facilitated in part by the developmental relevancy of the issues he was addressing. Self psychological views on adolescence (Kohut, 1987; Wolf, 1980b, 1982; Wolf, Gedo, & Terman, 1972) emphasize transformation and firming of the self as the major developmental task. Peers, in particular, take on special importance during this period, as relationships with parental selfobjects are redefined. The adolescent must move toward choosing "the vocation, the companions, the milieu, and the paths and ideals which will be available to function as selfobjects in supporting the self's cohesion" (Wolf, 1982, p. 180) throughout adult life. In Jim's case, the maturation of realistic ambitions, increase in affect and tension regulation, and expansion of the selfobject milieu which he displayed are all in particular ascendancy as developmental tasks during late adolescence. The press of these developmental demands undoubtedly contributed to his dramatic improvement in each of these areas, once the establishment of a selfobject bond with the therapist enabled him to reinstate the forward momentum of this developmental process.

For many people, a loss of requisite selfobject experiences is the precipitating and destabilizing event that weakens the self and leads to a search for therapy. Self psychology offers a particularly useful framework for understanding how cohesion and vitality can be restored in such cases, by use of the therapist as a selfobject for repair.

Certainly, many people need more. It has been my experience, however, that among a general population of people presenting themselves for help at a community clinic, a substantial number can be helped significantly in time-limited therapy when the central focus of the therapist's efforts is on the repair or restoration of the patient's sense of self-esteem, vigor and self-cohesion. Jim's case goes further, illustrating how in some cases the patient can go beyond repair and use even a brief treatment relationship to reinstate a process of development and structure building. Jim's age and relative health undoubtedly facilitated this outcome. Nevertheless, I have been repeatedly surprised at how many people of all ages and levels of pathology have been able to make good use of treatment conducted along these lines.

There is much work to be done to clarify both how to maximize therapeutic effectiveness when time is limited and how to identify those patients who are most apt to benefit from the kind of brief psychotherapy described here. In terms of the latter, self psychology appears potentially more promising than a number of previously developed brief psychodynamic therapies, where the selection criteria are so narrow as to exclude a majority of the patients who apply.

In practical terms, the time limitations on psychotherapy are determined much more by extrinsic factors than by the theoretical orientations of psychotherapists. It is most often clinic policies, third-party reimbursement parameters or the patient's own financial and emotional limitations that dictate how long the patient and therapist will have to work together. Increasingly, that period of time is fixed and it is brief. As therapists, we are left with the challenge of how best to use the time we have so as to maximally help our patients. I believe that brief psychotherapy is an eminently appropriate domain for the application of self psychology and that self psychology, in turn, holds great promise for enhancing the effectiveness of brief psychotherapy.

Notes

1 An extended description of this case was later published by the therapist P. Ornstein (1988).
2 The earlier work of Balint, P. Ornstein, and Balint (1972) and of P. Ornstein and A. Ornstein (1972) on focal psychotherapy, although not expressed in the language of contemporary self psychology, had underscored the functions of the therapist–patient relationship as a critical dimension of the mutative process.
3 I am very grateful to Jim's therapist, Betty Contorer, for providing the detailed case material that follows.

References

Bacal, H. (1985). Optimal responsiveness and the therapeutic process. In A. Goldberg (Ed.), *Progress in self psychology* (Vol. 1, pp. 202–227). New York, NY: Guilford.

Bacal, H. (1990). The elements of a corrective selfobject experience. *Psychoanalytic Inquiry*, *10*, 347–372.

Bacal, H., & Newman, K. (1990). *Theories of object relations: Bridges to self psychology.* New York, NY: Columbia University Press.

Balint, M., Ornstein, P., & Balint, E. (1972). *Focal psychotherapy: An example of applied psycho-analysis.* London, UK: Tavistock.

Basch, M.F. (1980). *Doing psychotherapy.* New York, NY: Basic Books.

Basch, M.F. (1988). *Understanding psychotherapy: The science behind the art.* New York, NY: Basic Books.

Budman, S. (Ed.). (1981). *Forms of brief therapy.* New York, NY: Guilford.

Chernus, L. (1983). Focal psychotherapy and self pathology: A clinical illustration. *Clinical Social Work Journal*, *11*, 215–227.

Donovan, J. (1987). Brief dynamic psychotherapy: Toward a more comprehensive model. *Psychiatry*, *50*, 167–183.

Elson, M. (1986). *Self psychology in clinical social work.* New York, NY: Norton.

Gardner, J.R. (1991). The application of self psychology to brief psychotherapy. *Psychoanalytic Psychology*, *8*, 477–500.

Goldberg, A. (1973). Psychotherapy of narcissistic injuries. *Archives of General Psychiatry*, *28*, 722–726.

Goldberg, A. (Ed.). (1978). *The psychology of the self: A casebook.* New York, NY: International Universities Press.

Goldberg, A. (Ed.). (1980a). *Advances in self psychology.* New York, NY: International Universities Press.

Goldberg, A. (1980b). Self psychology and the distinctiveness of psychotherapy. *International Journal of Psychoanalytic Psychotherapy*, *8*, 57–70.

Goldberg, A. (Ed.). (1983). *The future of psychoanalysis.* New York, NY: International Universities Press.

Goldberg, A., & Stepansky, P. (Eds.). (1984). *Kohut's legacy.* Hillsdale, NJ: The Analytic Press.

Kohut, H. (1959). Introspection, empathy and psychoanalysis. *Journal of the American Psychoanalytic Association*, *7*, 459–483.

Kohut, H. (1966). Forms and transformations of narcissism. *Journal of the American Psychoanalytic Association*, *14*, 243–272.

Kohut, H. (1971). *The analysis of the self.* New York, NY: International Universities Press.

Kohut, H. (1977). *The restoration of the self.* New York, NY: International Universities Press.

Kohut, H. (1978). The psychoanalyst in the community of scholars. In P. Ornstein (Ed.), *The search for the self* (pp. 685–724). New York, NY: International Universities Press. (Original work published 1973)

Kohut, H. (1982). Introspection, empathy, and the semi-circle of mental health. *International Journal of Psychoanalysis*, *63*, 395–407.

Kohut, H. (1984). *How does analysis cure?* Chicago, IL: University of Chicago Press.

Kohut, H. (1987). *The Kohut seminars on self psychology and psychotherapy with adolescents and young adults* (M. Elson, Ed.). New York, NY: Norton.

Kohut, H., & Wolf, E.S. (1978). Disorders of the self and their treatment. *International Journal of Psychoanalysis, 59*, 413–425.

Lazarus, L. (1980). Brief psychotherapy of narcissistic disturbances. *Psychotherapy: Theory, Research and Practice, 19*, 228–236.

Lazarus, L. (1988). Self psychology: Its application to brief psychotherapy with the elderly. *Journal of Geriatric Psychiatry, 21*, 109–125.

Miller, J. (1991). Can psychotherapy substitute for psychoanalysis? In A. Goldberg (Ed.), *The evolution of self psychology: Progress in self psychology* (Vol. 7, pp. 45–58). Hillsdale, NJ: The Analytic Press.

Ornstein, A. (1986). "Supportive" psychotherapy: A contemporary view. *Clinical Social Work Journal, 14*, 14–30.

Ornstein, A., & Ornstein, P. (1986). Empathy and the therapeutic dialogue. In *The Lydia Rappaport lecture series* (pp. 3–16). Northampton, MA: Smith School of Social Work.

Ornstein, P. (1988). Multiple curative factors and processes in the psychoanalytic psychotherapies. In A. Rothstein (Ed.), *How does treatment help?* (Workshop Series of the American Psychoanalytic Association, Monograph 4, pp. 105–126). Madison, CT: International Universities Press.

Ornstein, P., & Ornstein, A. (1972). Focal psychotherapy: Its potential impact on psychotherapeutic practice in medicine. *Journal of Psychiatry in Medicine, 3*, 311–325.

Ornstein, P., & Ornstein, A. (1977). On the continuing evolution of psychoanalytic psychotherapy: Reflections and predictions. *The Annual of Psychoanalysis, 5*, 329–370.

Socarides, D., & Stolorow, R. (1984–1985). Affects and selfobjects. *The Annual of Psychoanalysis, 12/13*, 105–119.

Stolorow, R. (1983). Self psychology—A structural psychology. In J.D. Lichtenberg & S. Kaplan (Eds.), *Reflections on self psychology* (pp. 287–296). Hillsdale, NJ: The Analytic Press.

Stolorow, R. (1986). Critical reflections on the theory of self psychology: An inside view. *Psycho-analytic Inquiry, 6*, 387–402.

Terman, D. (1988). Optimum frustration: Structuralization and the therapeutic process. In A. Goldberg (Ed.), *Learning from Kohut: Progress in self psychology* (Vol. 4, pp. 113–126). Hillsdale, NJ: The Analytic Press.

Terman, D. (1989). Therapeutic change: Perspectives of self psychology. *Psychoanalytic Inquiry, 9*, 88–100.

Tolpin, M. (1971). On the beginnings of a cohesive self. *The Psychoanalytic Study of the Child, 26*, 316–352.

Tolpin, M. (1983). Corrective emotional experience: A self psychological reevaluation. In A. Goldberg (Ed.), *The future of psychoanalysis* (pp. 363–380). New York, NY: International Universities Press.

Tolpin, P. (1985). The primacy of the preservation of the self. In A. Goldberg (Ed.), *Progress in self psychology* (Vol. 1, pp. 83–87). New York, NY: Guilford.

Tolpin, P. (1988). Optimal affective engagement: The analyst's role in therapy. In A. Goldberg (Ed.), *Learning from Kohut: Progress in self psychology* (Vol. 4, pp. 160–167). Hillsdale, NJ: The Analytic Press.

Tolpin, P. (1991). Analytic psychotherapy and psychoanalysis: A continuum? In A. Goldberg (Ed.), *The evolution of self psychology: Progress in self psychology* (Vol. 7, pp. 59–64). Hillsdale, NJ: The Analytic Press.

Winnicott, D.W. (1958). Transitional objects and transitional phenomena. In *Collected papers* (pp. 229–242). London, UK: Tavistock. (Original work published 1951)

Wolf, E.S. (1980a). On the developmental line of selfobject relations. In A. Goldberg (Ed.), *Advances in self psychology* (pp. 117–130). New York, NY: International Universities Press.

Wolf, E. (1980b). Tomorrow's self: Heinz Kohut's contribution to adolescent psychiatry. *Adolescent Psychiatry, 8*, 41–50.

Wolf, E. (1982). Adolescence: Psychology of the self and selfobjects. *Adolescent Psychiatry, 10*, 171–181.

Wolf, E.S. (1988). *Treating the self: Elements of clinical self psychology.* New York, NY: Guilford.

Wolf, E., Gedo, J., & Terman, D. (1972). On the adolescent process as a transformation of the self. *Journal of Youth and Adolescence, 1*, 257–272.

Chapter 3

Practical Steps for Using Self Psychology in Brief Treatment

This chapter duplicates parts of the ground covered in the previous chapter, but approaches and expands the ideas presented there through different vehicles. Rather than an extended clinical case, a series of organizing questions and frameworks is provided to facilitate the clinician's capacity to apply a self psychological point of view to the understanding and conduct of brief treatment. The goal of this piece is to elaborate on some of the practical steps involved in translating the theory into practice. How to conceptualize a case and how to look at patient selection, treatment planning, symptoms, adaptations, strengths and termination, among other topics, are areas described and illustrated with brief examples.

This paper was published in 1999 as "Using Self Psychology in Brief Psychotherapy" in Psychoanalytic Social Work, *Volume 6.*

Brief or time-limited psychotherapy is not usually seen as the province of self psychology, a theory which emerged in the context of psychoanalysis. Yet, as described previously (Gardner, 1991), I believe that brief psychotherapy is an eminently appropriate and fertile domain for the application of self psychology and that self psychology, in turn, can greatly enhance the effectiveness of brief treatment.

In this form of treatment, the therapist attends centrally to the state of the patient's self and the establishment of a selfobject bond with the therapist as a matrix for change. The core mutative process occurs through empathic interpretations which articulate and legitimize the patient's subjective experience, particularly his or her frustrated selfobject needs and longings. This process strengthens the self, leading to a reorganization of experience and reinstating a process of development, repair and structure building. All of these events can and do occur even in the context of very time-limited therapeutic encounters.

DOI: 10.4324/9781003491453-4

The goal of the present chapter is to elaborate some of the practical steps involved in the application of this theoretical perspective. I address this goal primarily by providing a set of questions and organizing frameworks, intended to help clinicians conceptualize brief treatment from a self psychological point of view. Before turning to this material, I offer a revised and updated review of the summary of self psychology theory and literature on brief treatment presented in my earlier article (Gardner, 1991).[1]

The Psychology of the Self: A Summary

Basic Concepts

The theory of self psychology, as developed originally by Kohut (1966, 1971, 1977, 1984; Kohut & Wolf, 1978) and his followers, provides an integrated view of normal development, psychopathology and the treatment process.

Kohut defined the core of development as the maturation of a cohesive nuclear self, imbued with basic strivings for power and success, basic idealized goals, and basic talents and skills (Kohut & Wolf, 1978). This self is developed and sustained by the empathic response of others who meet lifelong needs for validation, borrowed strength and a sense of belonging.

The developing child has a need for admiring and confirming responses to his or her innate sense of vigor and greatness. With appropriate validation or mirroring, this early expansiveness matures into self-esteem, assertiveness, ambition, a healthy enjoyment of successes and pleasure in the pursuit of interests and activities.

The child also has a need for closeness and support from an omnipotent source of calmness and strength. When the child is permitted to merge with the idealized calmness and strength of parental figures, these needs are transformed into ideals and values, idealized goals, and respect and admiration for others. Transformation of early idealizing needs also leads to the capacity for self-soothing, self-comfort and self-regulation, particularly in regard to affect and tension states.

Finally, Kohut defined a basic need for twinship as the reassuring experience of essential alikeness, belonging and kinship with others. He saw appropriate human closeness and twinship or alter-ego experiences as leading to a capacity to utilize optimally one's talents and skills.

The emergence of the self requires the presence of others who provide experiences that will evoke and maintain the self's cohesion (Wolf, 1988). These are called selfobject experiences. Selfobject refers to the internal, subjective experience of functions provided by others who are experienced as a needed part of the self (Wolf, 1988). The functions Kohut described were mirroring, idealizing and alter-ego experiences. More recently, Lichtenberg (1991) emphasized that the term "selfobject" refers less to a function than to "a vitalizing affective experience," crucial for maintaining a cohesive and vital sense of self.

Although these ideas were initially developed in the context of Kohut's work with narcissistically disordered patients, they were expanded by Kohut and others into a general theory of human motivation and development. Self psychology holds that the guiding force in human development is the need for connections to sources of selfobject experiences throughout life. The forms that these experiences take change as selfobject relations mature (Wolf, 1980), but the needs do not go away. Kohut considered this to be a fundamental theoretical shift from the centrality of instinctual, biological drives to the motivational primacy of self experience, that is, the psychological need for a milieu of empathic selfobjects from birth to death (Kohut, 1984).

The adequacy of the early selfobject milieu in meeting the child's developmental needs determines the fate of the emerging self. The self crystallizes in the matrix of a particular selfobject environment through a process of psychological structure formation Kohut called transmuting internalization. In this process, selfobject functions initially provided by others are internalized to become self functions, or inner psychic structure. Structure means having formerly external functions permanently in one's possession (Kohut, 1987). These functions or capacities include self-righting, self-soothing, self-regulation and the maintenance of self-cohesion (M. Tolpin, 1971, 1983). With the acquisition of psychic structure, the self grows cohesive and firm.

Structure can also be described in terms of how experience becomes increasingly organized, through the empathic response of parents to the child's affect. As Stolorow (1998) put it, the concept of selfobject function emphasizes that "the organization of self-experience is co-determined by the felt responsiveness of others" (p. 7). Through early interactions of mutual influence between parent and child, the child develops expectancies regarding interactional patterns (Beebe & Lachmann, 1988). These patterns of interaction are then internalized to become part of the inner structure and regulatory capacities of the child (Elson, 1989). Thus, structure also refers to these "invariant organizing principles" (Stolorow & Atwood, 1992) which shape the child's inner world.

When the process of structuralization is incomplete, one's self experience is vulnerable to a loss of cohesion or vitality in the face of selfobject failure. A variety of narcissistic injuries, separations or disruptions in relationships can precipitate the loss of requisite selfobject experience. This leads to fragmentation, enfeeblement, rage and various measures to maintain or restore the integration of self experience and a subjective sense of well being.

The origin of psychopathology lies in disturbances in the self-selfobject relations of childhood. When the child's need for empathic responsiveness is not adequately met by caregivers, development becomes derailed, leading to structural deficits and pathological defenses. The latter are erected to safeguard or restore the fragile self and to prevent further fragmentation or traumatization. The resulting self disorder reflects an inability to regulate affect and self-esteem, pursue meaningful goals, or express and meet needs in mature and age-appropriate forms. The problem is not one of conflict, as in classical libido theory, but of deficit: Normal development has been derailed and needs to be resumed.

Thus, treatment involves strengthening or rehabilitating the self. Kohut (1984) described the outcome of successful treatment in terms of both an increase in internal structure, reflected in greater firmness, cohesion and vigor of the patient's self, and an expansion of the patient's selfobject milieu, reflected in an increasing ability to identify, seek out and be sustained by appropriate selfobject experiences (both mirroring and idealizing), as currently available.

Placing more emphasis on the reorganization of experience, Fosshage (1998) described therapy as leading to new ways of organizing the sense of self, others and relationships. Treatment outcomes also include expansion of awareness and improved capacities for self-righting (Lichtenberg, Lachmann, & Fosshage, 1992, 1996).

Therapeutic Processes

Kohut consistently emphasized the importance of looking at the patient's experience from the patient's own perspective. The therapist gains access to this experience by the process of empathy, defined as "vicarious intro-spection" (Kohut, 1959, 1984). Empathy is a mode of observation which enables the therapist to grasp the affective state of the patient "while simultaneously retaining the stance of an objective observer" (Kohut, 1984, p. 175).

The therapist speaks to the patient's subjective experience and internal reality, communicating what he or she understands the patient to be saying. In this process, the therapist helps the patient to organize and clarify the meaning of his or her experience, while underscoring the salient feelings in the patient's statements. In particular, the therapist aims to articulate an empathic understanding and acceptance of the underlying needs, wishes and longings which the patient's behavior reflects.

This way of responding enhances the patient's sense of the validity of his or her own experience. Kohut believed that faulty empathy in the past leads to a repudiation of needs which interferes with getting them met in the present. What is unacceptable to caregivers must be defensively warded off in order to protect the selfobject bond and, ultimately, the self, whose well being is contingent on that bond. In contrast, when the therapist shares his or her sense of the legitimacy of the patient's needs, it facilitates the patient's ability to integrate and transform them into their mature counter-parts (Kohut, 1984).

The empathic mode of listening and responding makes contact with the patient's inner experience, enlivening his or her communications and engaging the patient in a "therapeutic dialogue" (A. Ornstein & Ornstein, 1986). The therapist's empathic responsiveness also creates an ambience and sense of safety that facilitate the patient's sharing and exploring previ-ously repressed or disavowed aspects of experience, which formerly were too threatening to permit awareness. Once these become part of the dia-logue, the therapist is in a position to offer the patient empathic interpreta-tions of them. Such interpretations bring relief by virtue of their "giving meaning to otherwise frightening and bewildering affects and thoughts" (P. Ornstein & Ornstein, 1977, p. 349).

Wolf (1988) described how the ambience created in this process can lead to the resumption of development:

> ... the accepting ambience of being in the presence of a respected per-son who is seriously, nonjudgmentally, and empathically interested in the patient's inner world may be the first such experience in their life.

Treatment becomes the first occasion to be in a milieu that facilitates the healing of the self by allowing those aspects of the self which had been arrested in their development to resume developing.

(p. 109)

This process occurs through the therapy relationship. Kohut (1984) described the reactivation of thwarted developmental needs as the essential driving force of the treatment process. As Elson (1986) elaborated, the therapist, functioning as a new source of selfobject experience and responding to the patient's emerging transference needs, reactivates development at the point at which earlier attempts to secure appropriate response from selfobjects failed. The patient's selfobject demands are viewed as legitimate expressions of his or her wish for the therapist to perform missing intrapsychic functions. In response to the patient's search for responses to these legitimate needs for structure building, the therapist becomes a source of selfobject functions that can be transmuted into the patient's own functional capacities, or inner psychic structure.

When the problem that brings the patient to treatment reflects a loss of previously established cohesion or vigor due to narcissistic injury or other disruptions in the selfobject milieu, the therapist similarly responds to the patient's selfobject needs in ways which allow the patient to restore his or her self to the previous level of functioning. For many people, a loss of requisite selfobject experiences is the precipitating and destabilizing event which weakens the self and leads to a search for therapy. Self psychology offers a particularly useful framework for understanding how cohesion and vitality can be restored in such cases, by use of the therapist as a selfobject for repair.

It is not that the therapist actively tries to put himself or herself in the role of selfobject; rather, it is the spontaneous transference of the patient's needs onto the therapist which puts the therapist in this role (M. Tolpin, 1983). When the therapist is then optimally responsive to these needs, which have arisen out of deficits in prior selfobject relationships, a corrective or therapeutic selfobject experience occurs (Bacal, 1990).

Kohut (1959, 1984) defined empathy primarily as a mode of observation, a way of gathering the data needed to make interpretations. It was the understanding and explanation of disruptions in the selfobject transference bond with the therapist that he saw as transforming a potential trauma into an experience of "optimal frustration" and leading to the accretion of psychic structure.

Contemporary self psychologists place more emphasis on optimal responsiveness (Bacal, 1985, 1990, 1998) than optimal frustration and on the mutative value of the relationship itself. Terman (1988, 1989) described how the empathic bond with the therapist and the patient's experience of being understood are intrinsic parts of structure formation and the curative process. Terman argued that being understood is growth producing in its own right. The experience of the relationship with the therapist as different in significant ways from the relationships of childhood facilitates both the growth of new structure and the change of existing structure. In this process, previously thwarted developmental tendencies are able to resume in the context of an appropriate, facilitating response. Stolorow (1986) similarly described the therapeutic relationship as a "facilitating medium," which reinstates developmental processes of self-articulation and self-demarcation that had been previously aborted or arrested.

For Bacal (1990, 1998), therapy "cures" through a corrective selfobject experience, mediated via optimal responsiveness. Optimal responsiveness includes the therapist's communications which "that particular patient experiences as usable for the cohesion, strengthening, and growth of his self. That is, the analyst's communications that are therapeutic are experienced by the patient as the provision of selfobject functions" (1990, p. 361).

More recently, the concept of a "positive new experience" (Shane, Shane, & Gales, 1997), going beyond empathy and interpretation, has been introduced to define a range of interventions which certain patients require in order to experience a selfobject connection with the therapist.

Integrating these different threads, Fosshage (1998) defined the goals of treatment as being achieved through a combination of ongoing selfobject experience, analysis of ruptures in the therapy relationship, illumination of problematic organizing patterns, and new relational experiences with the therapist. It is the latter which enables the patient to develop new representational schemata.

In these more recent conceptualizations, change is described more in terms of the reorganization and integration of affect than the acquisition of structure. Socarides and Stolorow (1984–1985) saw the integration and transformation of affect, leading to increases in both affect tolerance and articulation, as a central task of treatment. Even more pointedly, Basch (1988, 1995) defined affect management as the essence of psychotherapy.

Brief Treatment and Self Psychology

The rather extensive literature on short-term, dynamic psychotherapy contains relatively few articles written explicitly from a self psychological perspective. Books by Basch (1980, 1988, 1992), Kohut (1987) and Elson (1986) and an article by A. Ornstein and P. Ornstein (1996), though not about short-term psychotherapy *per se*, do include a number of brief treatment cases which were informed by the authors' self psychological perspective. They provide, for this reason, useful illustrative material.

Although he did not explicitly write about short-term therapy, Kohut (1987) saw his ideas as very relevant for brief treatment. He felt that a little bit of help, emanating from the borrowed strength of the therapist's support, could accomplish a great deal.

Goldberg (1973) offered perhaps the earliest explicit attempt to apply the evolving insights of self psychology to short-term psychotherapy. Discussing the psychotherapeutic treatment of narcissistic injuries, he described a need for the patient to be able to use the therapist as a source of selfobject functions in order to restore self-esteem. It was specifically in the understanding and interpretation of the patient's frustrated selfobject longings that repair of the injured self was seen to occur.

Like Goldberg, Lazarus (1980) conceptualized the goal of brief therapy with narcissistic disturbances as one of reestablishing the patient's feelings of self-esteem and self-cohesion by allowing the patient to use the therapist as a source of selfobject experience. He saw the reinstatement of the patient's pre-morbid level of functioning as the primary outcome in most cases. However, he also believed that in some cases the patient might begin to internalize the therapist's functions, leading to an accretion of psychic structure and further working through of narcissistic problems after termination.

In a later paper, Lazarus (1988) described the use of self psychological principles to conduct brief psychotherapy with elderly patients whose entry into treatment was precipitated by a narcissistic injury or other selfobject loss. Lazarus again described how the relationship with the empathic therapist may serve as a bridge to restore self-esteem and enable the patient to reestablish a supportive selfobject milieu outside of the treatment context.

Chernus (1983) described the use of focal psychotherapy (a close precursor of this model) to treat a structural deficit in the self, thus expanding the terrain previously described by others. In the case she reported, the *primary*

therapeutic goals were structure building and internalization of the therapist's selfobject functions, rather than the repair of the self and return to the
pre-morbid levels of functioning which had been emphasized by previous
authors. (For an extended description of this case, see the report later published by the therapist, P. Ornstein, 1988.)

Chernus also suggested that the briefer the treatment, the more likely
it was that the weight of the working-through process would occur in the
context of the patient's external relationships and experiences, rather than
in the transference to the therapist. P. Ornstein and A. Ornstein (1972) similarly found that working through occurred in meaningful ways outside of
the therapeutic relationship.

In a detailed case report, Gardner (1991) also described a process of
structural change occurring through brief, self psychological treatment.
Baker (1991) published a paper around the same time which similarly sum-
marized how self psychological principles could guide brief psychotherapy.

Taking a different approach, Ringstrom (1995) used a combination
of intersubjectivity theory (Stolorow, Brandchaft, & Atwood, 1987) and
motivational systems theory (Lichtenberg, 1989) to suggest a new model
of brief treatment. His focus was on the uncovering and modification of
unconscious organizing principles, emerging in the intersubjective context
of the transference relationship and illuminated through the analysis of
paradigmatic model scenes (Lichtenberg et al., 1992). He also emphasized
the importance of self-state assessment, a concept which is elaborated on at
length later in the present chapter.

A major addition to the literature appeared with the publication of
Basch's (1995) book on brief psychotherapy. One of Kohut's closest
original collaborators, Basch integrated, applied and extended the major
developments in self psychology, creating a developmental model which
emphasized affect while integrating cognition and information processing.
Major emphasis was placed on the mobilization of the patient's strengths to
facilitate brief treatment.

Finally, Seruya (1997) offered a model of "empathic brief psychotherapy," which integrated self psychology with cognitive-behavioral theory.
While not exclusively self psychological in approach, her model draws on
self psychology extensively, provides an excellent summary of the theory
and extends the model to brief work with couples.

Although the literature on self psychology and brief psychotherapy is not
extensive, it is encouraging that it is increasing. As stated earlier, I believe

that brief psychotherapy is fertile ground for the application of self psychology, which, in turn, can make brief psychotherapy more effective.

The concepts described above provide a conceptual roadmap for self psychologically informed brief treatment. However, the exact way these concepts are applied is not always clear to those who seek to practice this model. In the sections below, I address this issue by describing some pragmatic steps to assist clinicians in making the translation from theory to practice.

It is also important to note that there is not one approach to brief treatment within self psychology, but many. The literature just reviewed provides a variety of viewpoints regarding what we do, how we do it and why it works. My own approach draws most heavily on the contributions of Basch and the Ornsteins, along with my experience doing and supervising brief treatment in the settings of a hospital-based, community mental health center and private practice. The model I describe is not a particular technique, but rather a series of components which, when put together, make treatment more efficient and briefer.

Patient Selection

Most approaches to brief therapy prescribe selection criteria. It is certainly logical to begin by trying to determine whether a given patient is a suitable candidate for self psychologically informed brief treatment. Yet this begs the question that most clinicians face. In some settings, patients can indeed be directed to brief or open-ended treatment tracks at an intake level. In most cases, however, it is not the therapist but rather clinic policies, third-party reimbursement parameters or the patient's own financial, time and emotional limitations that dictate how long the patient and therapist will have to work together. When the length of the treatment is set arbitrarily by these extrinsic factors, the question becomes less one of who is appropriate and more one of how to use whatever time one has. Bellak (Bellak & Small, 1978) reflected this reality when he suggested that what we select, essentially, is problems and goals, not patients.

Another stumbling block to using well-established selection criteria is the lack of empirical data upon which to base them. Early models of brief dynamic treatment did have good outcome studies (see Messer & Warren, 1995, for a comprehensive review) but were criticized for using selection criteria which were so narrow as to exclude a majority of the patients who applied. A more recent approach (Basch, 1995), taking the opposite stance, suggests that we consider *all* patients as potentially suitable candidates for brief dynamic treatment until proven otherwise. How do we prove otherwise? Are there prognostic clues we can rely on? Fortunately, the lack of systematic outcome studies has not kept theorists from offering some suggestions.

A. Ornstein and P. Ornstein (1997) saw their capacity to formulate a focus early on as a key determinant for successful brief treatment. For the Ornsteins, a focus is not the presenting problem but a formulation that *explains* the presenting problem. Whether or not the therapist can arrive quickly at such an organizing formulation and focus the treatment around it is seen as a crucial prognostic indicator.

Ringstrom (1995) believed that the rapidity with which someone has a positive response to the therapist's empathy may be a good predictor of the efficacy of brief treatment. Drawing on Lichtenberg et al.'s (1992) observation that the state of the self depends on a person's responsiveness to empathy and vulnerability to lack of empathy, he urged therapists to consider questions such as: How restorative or fragmenting are the first sessions? How responsive is the patient to the therapist's attunement?

Most clinicians have had the experience of offering an empathic connection which is like water to a wilted plant for one patient and water off a duck's back to another. The former seems to grow firmer before our eyes, while the latter stares at us blankly, seeming to ignore whatever we say. Others respond aversively, with antagonism, withdrawal or anxiety.

Basch (1995) emphasized the presence of an idealizing transference, stating that the success of brief treatment may depend on whether a positive (idealizing) transference is in place or can quickly be mobilized.

> Indeed, the question of whether or not short term therapy can be effective or whether lengthier treatment is needed depends often not so much on the nature of the problem *per se*, but on how soon patients can permit themselves to feel safe, supported, and enhanced in the therapeutic relationship.
>
> (p. 94)

When Basch used the term "idealization," he was referring to the patient's capacity to rely on the therapist's guidance and support.[2] This is a necessary prerequisite for both trust and credibility; if the patient can't idealize or rely on the therapist, validation or mirroring from that therapist won't have any impact. Validation which is useful to us has to come from credible sources whom we can look up to in some fashion.

Basch also underscored how patients who are highly defended or resistant often require longer treatment to work through their shame over needing to rely on the therapist before any progress can be made. Because shame interferes with letting needs arise in therapy, it must be sufficiently resolved before the patient can tolerate both the therapeutic relationship and the underlying painful affects which have been protectively warded off (Basch, 1988, 1995; Kohut, 1984). It is through the vicissitudes and analysis of the transference that such patients' problems eventually become manifest and are resolved.

There were two other groups of people whom Basch defined as usually *not* good candidates for brief treatment: people who need to make up for substantial developmental deficits and those needing prolonged support in order to function. He didn't believe that brief therapy could be a substitute for dealing with these problems in more open-ended treatment. At the same time, he saw people needing long-term psychoanalysis or long-term support as being at the ends of the bell curve, leaving a lot of people in the middle. He was fond of saying, "When all you have is a hammer, everything looks like a nail" (Basch, 1995, p. xii). By this he meant that it was our attachment to psychoanalysis and lack of alternative methodologies that led to our reluctance to realize that brief treatment might be the treatment of choice for many of our patients.

My own experience is that many people can work in circumscribed problem areas, leave major domains of character pathology untouched and derive considerable benefit from relatively brief treatment. Others can reinstate a process of structural growth and change, impacting long-standing patterns. (For case illustrations of the latter, see Chernus [1983] and Gardner [1991], in addition to Basch [1995].)

The more conventional clinical indicators we usually consider in evaluating patients for brief treatment remain important: How pervasive the problems are, how limited, how long they have been going on, the presence of clear precipitants, the extent of substance abuse and the degree of other internal resources and external supports, to name a few. But, having been both surprised and wrong often enough, I have come to believe that it is more useful to begin with the assumption that the patient in front of us could potentially benefit from brief treatment and then look for what, if anything, would lead us to disconfirm that assumption. It might be severe, uncontrolled substance abuse; it might be massive defenses against enough idealization to make at least some use of what the therapist has to offer. It might become obvious in the first ten minutes, or it might take several sessions to determine.

Self psychologists, warning against the dangers of selectively perceiving or molding data to fit our preconceived conceptual schemata, have begun to suggest that we should "hold our theories lightly" (Orange, 1995). When we approach the task of determining which patients might benefit from brief treatment, we would do well to hold our assumptions lightly as well.

Treatment Planning as a Clinical Process and Collaborative Activity

If what we select has more to do with *what* we work on than *whom* we work with, we need to turn our attention to how the relevant issues get selected. For many clinicians, the words treatment planning have come to signify onerous forms and administrative intrusion into the treatment process. Psychodynamic practitioners, in particular, often experience the idea of treatment planning as inimical to their way of working. Yet treatment planning is crucial to the success of brief treatment. What we need is another way to think about it.

I see treatment planning as evolving out of the clinical exploration of problems and goals, that is, as a clinical process not an administrative one. Treatment planning is a way of establishing an explicit understanding with the patient of the nature of why he or she is there and what's to be done. Most importantly, it involves engaging the patient as an active collaborator in defining the purpose of therapy.

Collaborative treatment planning reinforces the patient as a center of initiative in the therapy process. It promotes ownership and patient responsibility, helps to prioritize problems and facilitates the establishment of a focus. Basch (1995) noted that "the process of establishing what the patient is there to accomplish is in itself therapeutic" (p. 52). If we just listen to problems without also hearing what the patient expects to see as an outcome, we may hamper a short-term focus. Problems are not equivalent to goals. We also need to ask how the patients see therapy as helping or relevant to their presenting concerns. Questions regarding their view of what they need from us can be very helpful in clarifying the particular strengths they bring to the process, along with their difficulties.

The material which follows addresses, from several different perspectives, the issue of focusing the treatment, starting on a broadly conceptual level and then moving through some very specific ways of determining the issues to be worked on.

Central Focus on Self Experience and Selfobject Relationship with Therapist

In any kind of brief or time-limited treatment, the therapist must decide where to put his or her therapeutic energy, given limited resources. All forms of brief therapy address the issue of focus in one way or another. From a self psychological perspective, the therapist's central focus must be on the self experience of the patient and on the relationship between the patient and therapist as a new self-selfobject unit. This selfobject bond is the matrix in which change takes place. In brief treatment, as in longer term treatment, the emphasis is on strengthening the self.[3] When there has been a weakening or disorganization of self experience (manifested in decreased cohesion or vitality) due to changes and losses in the selfobject surround, then the selfobject relationship with the therapist functions as a bridge to restore the self to its previous healthier state.

Thus, whatever the specific precipitants, symptoms or treatment goals may be, the therapist must (a) attend specifically to ways in which the self is vulnerable, injured or arrested, (b) understand symptoms as manifestations of these deficits, and (c) enable the patient to establish the selfobject matrix required to facilitate repair and growth.

A. Ornstein (1986) suggested that concern with the state of the self should be the primary focus in the treatment of *all* patients, regardless of the nature of the pathology or form of the treatment. In any duration of treatment, feeling understood can lead to an increase in self-cohesion which allows an exploration of previously repressed or disavowed affects, wishes, fears and fantasies. The emergence of these previously unavailable aspects of the patient's experience into awareness provides an opportunity to understand their meaning and, in so doing, to use the therapy relationship to strengthen the self.

Elson (1986) stated it eloquently:

> Self psychology clarifies the universal striving to secure a response to one's potential for individuality and significance. In even the most seriously deprived individual, underneath abrasive and cynical behavior, a vestige of the need to be confirmed remains alive to be rekindled. The very presence of the [therapist] may quicken this need. Many methods and approaches have been devised for responding to and controlling the relationship which ensues, but, regardless of method, how one orders what one sees and experiences, how one uses oneself on behalf of the individual, becomes more vivid through an explanatory system of human behavior that places the self of the individual at the center of one's observations and views the new self/selfobject unit as the medium for treatment.
>
> (p. 136)

State of the Self

With the state of the self as a point of departure, assessment can be facilitated by a series of organizing questions which help both to conceptualize the clinical material and to establish a focus for treatment. These are described below under four broad headings: symptoms and deficits, adaptations, strengths and transference.

Symptoms and Deficits

There are two lenses through which a self psychologist might look at symptoms. The first asks: How do the patient's presenting symptoms express a deficit in, or loss of, the self's cohesion or vitality?

Patients who exhibit agitation, anxiety, disorganized behavior or a deterioration in appearance often signal through these symptoms a problem in the cohesiveness of their self experience. Incipient states of fragmentation are often characterized by debilitating disintegration anxiety (Tolpin & Kohut, 1980). One patient, usually meticulously groomed, arrived for her appointment in an agitated and disheveled state, saying that she felt "like humpty-dumpty." There is no more apt metaphor for fragmentation and the loss of cohesion than this nursery rhyme character who falls off a wall, splintering so irrevocably that "all the king's horses and all the king's men/ cannot put humpty together again."

The patient suffering from a lack or loss of vitality, in contrast, sags rather than splinters. When we see symptoms that cluster around a lack of energy, motivation and ambition, and the affect is melancholy, we think in terms of a devitalized or depleted sense of self.

Through the second lens on symptoms, we ask the question: In what ways do the patient's symptoms reflect attempts to restore or reorganize the weakened self? Substance abuse, eating disorders and sexual acting out may be used to stimulate and enliven someone with a sense of deadness or depletion. Any of these symptoms might also be employed to calm or reverse an anxious state of fragmentation. Some people get high to feel alive; others drink to calm their nerves. Some people overeat when they're anxious, others when they're bored and lonely. When we see an increase in any of these symptomatic behaviors, we can begin to think in terms of how the behavior reflects an attempt to alter the underlying self state the patient is experiencing. Attending specifically to the patient's subjective experience of the symptomatic behavior and its sequelae will usually clarify what that underlying self state is.

For example, a man who often felt slighted by his boss and coworkers would go cruising in bars for sex on days he suffered these narcissistic injuries. Although his dangerous promiscuity created other problems for him, the affirmation he found in being sexually desired helped restore his self-esteem and sense of vitality.

Another patient was driving her family and coworkers to distraction with her angry, irritable and controlling behavior. Her unreasonable attempts to force everyone to fulfill her minutest wishes could be understood as an effort to maintain eroding self-esteem and control over her selfobject world, as serious medical problems and job changes combined to make her feel totally out of control. This particular pattern of symptomatic behavior quite often is secondary to the sense of helplessness caused by illness, parenting problems or job-related stress.

Self psychologists generally view symptoms as the patient's best available means of protecting a fragile, vulnerable self against retraumatization or of revitalizing and reorganizing a depleted or fragmented self. Keeping these purposes in mind, we can ask the question: To what problem is this symptomatic behavior a solution? The answers help us make the translation from symptom to self state, an important step in determining the focus of treatment. It is a shift in understanding from the level of behavior, e.g., this person abuses cocaine, to the level of dynamics, e.g., this person has a crushing sense of deadness and he is devoid of other (internal) resources to counteract it. Symptoms reflect efforts to achieve both a reintegration on the level of self-organization and a shift in the subjective experience of self.

When we evaluate problematic affect, cognition and behavior, we also need to determine whether we are dealing with transient symptoms or ongoing deficits. Again, a series of questions is helpful: What deficits are apparent in the patient's self experience? Are they acute? Chronic? In other words, has this individual ever acquired the self-soothing and regulating functions needed to maintain self-esteem and regulate affect? To judge this, it would be helpful to know how prone the patient is to fragmentation or depletion experiences. Light could be shed on this by asking: Is the current upset less than, as bad as or worse than what the person has felt before? Is this a pretty typical way of feeling or is it unusual? As always, subjective experience is crucial. What one person considers an alarming sign of impending breakdown may for another be an everyday experience of self, albeit a painful or distressing one. To evaluate symptoms of anxiety or absent-mindedness, for example, it matters whether one is a person who is generally unflappable or one who is always worried, one who never misplaces things or one who can lose keys while holding them in their hand.

In a sense, I am discussing the pervasiveness and chronicity of presenting problems. Generally speaking, the more that symptoms reflect a *loss* of cohesion or vitality rather than a *lack* of them, the more likely it is that brief intervention may help the individual get back on course. Both Kohut (1987) and Elson (1986) offered several examples of this among student populations.

Adaptations

In conjunction with deficits, we also need to know: How, typically, has the person tried to compensate for these deficits? Here I am referring to the range of defensive adaptations, compensatory structures and characterological solutions which people devise, over the course of development, to deal with whatever trauma and selfobject failures they have experienced.

Most people have characteristic ways of coping, i.e., maintaining cohesion, competence or adaptive functioning, and avoiding anxiety. These ways of dealing with trouble and maintaining a viable sense of self include both internal mechanisms (functional capacities) and external supports (sources of needed selfobject experience).

The search for treatment is often precipitated by something which triggers an inability to cope. Usually the trigger is a loss or a new challenge. The situation then exposes what we might think of as "fault lines." These are structural deficits which are exposed when the usual defenses are overwhelmed. Precipitating stresses disrupt the previous adaptations and strain them to the point where they cannot hold. Although this development is often preceded by an initial redoubling of usual defensive efforts, these emergency measures eventually fail as well. It is at this point that the underlying problems may come more into view and can therefore become a focus of treatment.

For example, some people protect themselves against unbearable feelings of dependency by developing a pattern of defensive self-sufficiency. When external events, such as an accident, illness or job loss, necessitate requesting or accepting help from others, they become acutely anxious. The anxiety is associated with the memory of previous traumatic failures in the face of needs. It is the inability to employ the usual solution which reveals the underlying vulnerability. A more obvious example is phobic avoidance. As long as the object of one's phobia can be avoided, the patient appears asymptomatic. If the defense of avoidance is precluded or fails, however, the underlying anxiety immediately becomes apparent.

A similar problem can be observed in patients who rely on defensive isolation or distance to regulate their anxiety about intimacy. They often become symptomatic when external events necessitate more closeness than they are used to or comfortable with. Obvious examples are signs of increased commitment to a relationship, such as moving in with a partner, getting engaged or getting married. These are common times for us to see symptoms emerge. This problem can also be precipitated, however, by a change as innocuous seeming as needing to share an office at work. The loss of the physical wall or partition may subjectively constitute the loss of a psychological wall which enabled the person to function within a range of acceptable emotional distance.

One patient became increasingly anxious as her pregnancy progressed. Exploration revealed her ever-expanding abdomen as the focus of her distress. As we explored the meaning of this concern, she described her father's bitter disappointment in not having a son and his disdain for his two daughters. Desperately needing an antidote to her depressed mother, she managed to evoke some affirmation from her father by becoming a star athlete, winning a place on the national team in her sport. What her advancing pregnancy made clear was how her flat stomach had always been not only a source of pride, but a crucial symbol of the one thing that she felt made her valuable in the eyes of her father, securing the selfobject bond with him she urgently needed to maintain her self-esteem.

Sports and physical activity are often used to regulate tension, as well as self-esteem. It is not uncommon to see patients who rely on this outlet become both depressed and anxious when an injury prevents them from their usual routine. While others may simply become irritable or feel less energetic when they can't run or work out, for this kind of person more extensive underlying deficits in self-regulation become apparent.

The pressures in many workplaces brought about by downsizing and other cost-cutting measures create particular difficulty for people whose compulsivity and perfectionism are defensively tied to their psychological security. When one now has three jobs to cover, it is impossible to cover all the bases as thoroughly. A related pattern is the person who manages to stave off vulnerability and anxiety by being extremely competent, always on top of things. When external demands create more than anyone could humanly manage, no matter how skilled he or she is, the underlying vulnerability in self-esteem is revealed. It is usually the concurrence of several stressful events which triggers the problem in this type of individual.

Finally, and perhaps most prevalently, there is the person who must ward off affect to maintain his or her psychological equilibrium. It seems to matter less which particular defenses are used than it does that unmanageable (usually dysphoric) affect is kept at bay. When precipitating events mobilize too much affect to suppress, the person experiences emotional flooding, anxiety and symptoms. The characterological defenses against affect simply cannot handle the emotions which have been stimulated.

Some of these people say things like "I'm a coper," "I'm a minimizer" or "I'm a control freak." When something then happens which the person can't cope with, minimize or control, symptoms develop. It is often then not the presenting symptoms, or even the defenses, but rather the meaning of the need to minimize or control in the first place that becomes the focus of treatment. As the patient's usual means of sequestering underlying anxieties and affects fail, these experiences can be brought to light, understood and explained.

The conception of treatment I am elaborating here is very close to the model of focal psychotherapy developed by Balint and the Ornsteins (Balint, Ornstein, & Balint, 1972; P. Ornstein, 1988; P. Ornstein & Ornstein, 1972).

As defined by Chernus (1983), focal psychotherapy involves the exploration and working through of a focal conflict precipitated by a recent event which has overwhelmed the patient's characterological defense mechanisms. That characterological weakness becomes the focus of treatment. In contrast to the goal of crisis intervention, which is a return to the previous homeostasis, the goal of focal psychotherapy is a modification of the maladaptive defensive structures.

More recently, the Ornsteins (1997) have updated their description of brief focal psychotherapy in ways that clarify how the examination of symptoms, deficits and adaptations can create a focus in brief treatment. They suggest that, rather than trying to examine the whole personality, we should look at a slice or sector of the personality in depth. This look would cut across the levels of surface or presenting problems, attempts to cope with the problems, and core or nuclear problems. They emphasize that the current problem should make sense in terms of who the person has been for an entire life. In other words, the therapist must establish the dynamic connection between the current problem, precipitated by some kind of stress, and what has gone on in the person's life before. When such a formulation can be expressed in terms of an interpretive comment to the patient, it creates a focus for the treatment. As stated earlier, for the Ornsteins the focus is not the presenting problem, but rather a formulation which explains the presenting problem. Also, if the focus provides an explanation for the current problem while at the same time touching on the patient's character pathology, then work on the immediate problem includes working on the chronic problems.

Wolf (personal communication) expressed a similar idea by emphasizing that precipitating events often resonate with earlier events which have similar affective themes. It is these similarities which amplify the impact of the precipitating events and create continuity between past and present.

My own experience has been that successful cases of brief treatment often conform to these models. A woman referred by her employer because of the irritability and stress she was exhibiting at work reported a history of several recent medical problems, all quite serious. While she was aware of sadness and anger in connection with these problems, she was not in touch with her considerable anxiety. She only knew she was snapping at everyone around her. As she described her situation, she revealed herself to be a high-functioning, very competent person who characteristically downplayed both needs and dysphoric feelings. She said she was a "minimizer" who had "no tolerance for self-pity." However, as her sense of choice and control was being rapidly eroded by her health problems, she was confronted with feelings she could not successfully minimize, and her previous defenses no longer served to protect her from the anxiety such feelings created in her. Successful treatment focused on increasing her affect awareness and tolerance. When she could experience and express her feelings more directly, feeling entitled to them as legitimate, she regained her equilibrium and was able to terminate the treatment. I saw her a total of six times.

In another case, the patient came requesting help to better manage the tension associated with several external stresses in both his family and work life. His presenting complaint was depression. What quickly became apparent was his great difficulty in asserting himself effectively with a disabled relative who was making enormous demands on him. Although massively frustrated, he was trying very hard to be compassionate, understanding, tolerant and helpful. His history revealed that he had responded to a very critical and guilt-inducing parental environment with a combination of compliance, resentment and withdrawal. This was a man who had learned to sit on feelings until they reached a boiling point, at which point they felt too dangerous to express, leading him to retreat and to become depressed. Treatment focused on his long-standing fears regarding self-assertion. As with the previous case, effective treatment involved enabling him to identify and express his own needs and feelings more directly, even in the face of significant others in his life whose needs seemed to him much greater. It was this change in relation to his internal life that enabled him to achieve his original goal of managing the external stresses more effectively.

In both cases, it was a focus on the underlying problem in the self which was exposed by the failure of characteristic defenses that led to successful brief treatment. These cases also underscore Socarides and Stolorow's (1984–1985) emphasis on the central role of the selfobject transference bond in the "articulation, integration and developmental transformation of the patient's affectivity" (p. 112).

Strengths

When working with people in brief treatment, attention to their strengths becomes pivotal. We need to ask: What strengths are apparent in the patient's self experience and functioning? What has the patient used in the past to maintain or restore vitality and cohesion? Which self-restorative efforts have been helpful? In what areas does the patient continue to exhibit strength now?

Basch, in particular, emphasized the need to elicit and foster strengths and to focus on how the strengths no longer serve the patient, rather than focusing on the origins of problems in childhood. In his view, the patient is seen as possessing the resources to cope with his or her problem; the therapist's job is to mobilize them. He described the patient as an agent for change in the present rather than simply a victim of the past and saw patients' strengths as the leverage to help them do something about their problems (Basch, 1995).

> When we work successfully, we are not solving patients' problems *per se*; rather we are helping them to use or enhance what they have on the plus side to minimize, offset, and occasionally eradicate what is on the minus side. We are helping them to right themselves so that *they* will be in a position to solve the problems that brought them to us in the first place.
>
> (pp. 6–7)

Basch felt that people come to therapy because their strengths are no longer working. The fostering of self-righting, which he is describing above as a goal of treatment, has been emphasized by other self psychologists as well (Lichtenberg et al., 1992; M. Tolpin, 1983). Kohut actually talked 20 years earlier about mobilizing the patient's strengths. In a 1975 lecture he stated:

> In those cases in which the essential task is the analysis of a disturbed core self, the crucial work deal[s] predominantly with opening up the possibility of new choices ... with the freeing of sources of strength that were not present before ... the primary analytic task is understood to be an effort that will enable the patient to use something that is in him by freeing it or putting it in working order ... it is not that one is finally able to see that he has an unacceptable drive that has to be discarded, but that he has a central source of strength that was not available before.
>
> (Kohut, 1996, pp. 370–371)

Consistent with Kohut's, and later Basch's, emphasis on potentials for strength and growth, we need to emphasize what the person is doing right and support it. The orientation in our training toward pathology often interferes with this focus on strengths. A simple inquiry regarding what patients feel they need from us can be useful in supporting their capacities to define their own resources and limitations, reinforcing our view of them as active collaborators in the therapeutic endeavor.

On a practical level, Basch (1995) suggested that we note the content associated with shifts from negative to positive affect as the patient tells his or her story. He felt that such shifts toward brighter affect signal the hidden strengths and adaptive coping mechanisms one hopes to mobilize.

When the clinician then encourages an elaboration of the material following the shift, dramatic results can occur. One man had appeared in the first few sessions to be an inhibited and passive person, lacking drive or ambition, experiencing little pleasure in life and seeming drained rather than energized by his various activities. His presenting complaint was his inability to make commitments. In our conversations, he was formal, polite and subdued, often running out of things to say. However, when he began talking about a college friend he was reminded of by a dream, his face lit up with admiration and enthusiasm.

His obvious, vicarious enjoyment of his friend's wild antics and *joie de vivre*, in contrast to his own inhibited approach to life, led me to inquire whether there had ever been anything he felt he could put himself into fully. As he recalled an early artistic talent, his face again lit up. Guided by this shift in affect, I actively encouraged him to elaborate on things he had enjoyed. This revealed talents, creativity, imagination and humor which I could not have imagined he possessed and with which he, too, had long lost contact. The pleasure he experienced in remembering and sharing these more vibrant parts of himself marked a turning point in the treatment, seeming to infuse him with a newfound energy as he began to make decisions and actively take hold of his life.

Another man came to treatment with a crisis of confidence as he stood on the threshold of his professional career. He believed that only regaining a previously felt (and defensively held) sense of invincibility would cure his anxiety, inhibition and fear of competing in the marketplace. Hearing that he had been a soccer player, I asked him what he did when he was playing a game and fell down. With great emphasis, he replied, "I got up and got back in the game! If I gave up a goal, I was embarrassed, but then I tried even harder." This allowed me to suggest that perhaps what he had lost confidence in was not his invincibility, but his resiliency. Drawing on his history, I pointed out how over and over he had been able to turn an initial disappointment to advantage and move his life forward. Looking at this pattern helped him realize that even when he hadn't been invincible, he had nevertheless been successful. Armed with a new sense of confidence in his own resiliency, he became able to accept the much more attainable goal of "getting back in the game" following whatever setbacks might occur. With this shift, it took only a few sessions for him to come out of the malaise which had overtaken him and feel more secure about launching his career.

Sometimes the mobilization of strengths involves less reconnecting with previous experiences than reframing them. Basch (1995) was particularly effective at doing this. With one man who took his children's rather minor misconduct as disrespectful insults and challenges to his authority, complaining that *he* never behaved that way as a child, Basch replied that the man never had a chance to *be* a child, never behaved in all the ways that are typical of children and frustrating to adults. The fact that his kids could afford to do this was a compliment to what he had achieved psychologically for them. In contrast to his own, anxiety-filled childhood, his children had a basic confidence and trust that he would be there to take care of them, whether they responsibly performed every chore or not. Basch noted that this interpretation validates the patient's achievement, while protecting his fragile self-esteem. Reframing weakness to strength is a familiar process to self psychologists, who emphasize the adaptive and protective functions of behavior generally.

Transference Manifestations of Selfobject Needs

Manifestations of selfobject needs in the relationship with the therapist provide another way to understand the organization of self experience and state of the self. Insufficiently met selfobject needs lead to vulnerabilities in the self and defenses which are erected to protect the precariously organized self from retraumatization. When a patient enters therapy, the needs, vulnerabilities and defenses all become manifest in the transference. The unmet developmental needs are reflected in the "selfobject dimension" of the transference, while the vulnerabilities and defenses are reflected in the "repetitive/conflictual dimension" (Stolorow et al., 1987). Therefore, it is helpful to ask ourselves: What needs of the self are being expressed in the patient's behavior toward the therapist? What selfobject experiences is the patient appealing to us to be a source of? How are these manifested (or defended against)?

The patient who provides detailed descriptions of his activities and accomplishments, for example, may be seeking mirroring and validation through which to bolster self-esteem. The one who wants to "chat" may be searching for some kind of enlivening engagement with the therapist, not resisting deeper issues. A clamor for advice and direction may reflect an appeal to the therapist to be a source of idealizing selfobject functions which would organize and make sense out of the patient's experience. On the other hand, the patient who engages in hostile, provocative behavior toward the therapist may be trying to protect a vulnerable self from being retraumatized, by rejection or misunderstanding. Through behaviors which create distance and mask underlying vulnerabilities, the patient prevents exposure of previously thwarted selfobject needs. Kohut (1984) described this protective function as the fundamental goal of all defenses. When the therapist recognizes and affirms the legitimacy of whatever selfobject needs are evident in the transference, the self is strengthened. When the therapist fails to do so, the self is threatened and symptoms may worsen.

Careful attention to the selfobject dimension of the transference may also clarify the specific nature of underlying deficits or recent injuries, since patients tend to reactivate in the transference those selfobject needs which have been thwarted. In an early paper, Goldberg (1973) described two brief treatment cases who presented in nearly opposite ways to the therapist. The first patient "entered the hour as a storm-tossed and agitated man who wanted smoothing of his ruffled feathers and agreement and reflection of his outrage" (p. 724). The therapist was implicitly beseeched to admire the patient (his "charm, wit, and presence") and to refrain from any kind of criticism. In the second case, the patient immediately assigned to the therapist the role of an expert, who would tell him what was wrong with him and what to do about it.

These obvious bids to meet mirroring and idealizing needs, respectively, paralleled the internal meaning of the narcissistic injuries which had brought these patients to treatment. In the first case, the man became symptomatic after a group of students whom he had hoped to impress called him pompous; in the second, the patient's symptoms were triggered by his boss's failure to be the omnipotent protector for whom he longed.

By recognizing a patient's appeal in the transference for the therapist to be a source of reparative selfobject experiences, the therapist is alerted to the nature of the underlying difficulty. The specific problems which emerge through this process clarify deficits in the self and point to a potential focus for treatment. An analogous process for exploring precipitating events is described below.

As a final note regarding transference, it is important to reiterate the need to evaluate the extent to which a positive transference is either in place or is able to be mobilized quickly (cf. Basch, 1995). Even if more archaic needs emerge and are addressed, the therapist must be used for mature selfobject functions in the present, and this requires the idealization or reliance described earlier. When deeply entrenched defenses prevent such engagement, brief treatment may not be possible.

Subjective (internal) Meaning of Precipitating Events

All therapists seek to understand the role of precipitating events in the patient's presenting problems and search for treatment. This is the familiar question, "What brings you in now?" A self psychologically informed version of this question would ask: What is the meaning of the precipitating events in terms of their impact on the patient's self experience and selfobject surround? More specifically, how do the stresses which led the person to seek therapy involve the loss of important selfobject experiences? Which kinds of selfobject experiences were lost or became less available? And finally, what role did these experiences play in sustaining an inner sense of vitality and cohesion? All of these questions aim to clarify the nature of the *internal* problem that has to be addressed. As therapists, we respond not to external events, but to the subjective experience of those events. An empathic mode of inquiry is used to determine what the subjective experience is.

The internal loss might be precipitated by a loss or rupture in a relationship, leading to a temporary loss of cohesion, depletion or fragmentation. Or it may be precipitated by the loss of a role that was affirming, such as a job or parenting. Depending on the nature of the relationship or role, the selfobject experiences afforded might have met mirroring needs, such as the need for affirmation and appreciation, or idealizing ones, such as the availability of idealized strength and guidance.

When the normal process of psychic structure building is incomplete, an individual is more vulnerable to a loss of needed selfobject experiences. If a relationship is disrupted or ends, the selfobject loss is then more pronounced. For example, if the mirroring functions of a relationship were necessary to stabilize and maintain self-esteem, then with the other person could go the capacity to feel good about oneself. One patient, struggling with feelings about her physical appearance after breaking up with her boyfriend, expressed this very concretely:

> I miss the feedback I got from Perry. He always told me I looked good and made me feel attractive. Now I look in the mirror and I don't know what to think. I can't tell. I feel like I have to go to such effort to make myself look good and I don't always feel like it. But I would feel terrible if I went out and people saw me looking awful. With Perry, he just told me I looked good no matter what and I felt OK.

This description underscores the difficulty she is having regulating her self-esteem in the absence of her boyfriend's mirroring affirmation.

If, on the other hand, the calming and soothing functions of an idealized other are needed because of deficits in the person's own capacity for self-soothing, then with the loss of this selfobject dimension of the relationship may go the capacity for affect regulation and the ability to calm down. Increased anxiety and decreased cohesion usually follow. This is a very common pattern in patients with borderline personality disorders because of the extremely tenuous nature of their underlying self organization (P. Tolpin, 1984).

It becomes easier to understand how people stay in apparently destructive relationships when we consider these selfobject functions being served by them. A similar dynamic underlies the dissolution of relationships as well. As Wolf (1988) described:

> Much of the irritation of people with each other, the quarrels that tear up marriages, and the misunderstandings that lead to loss of spouse, friend, or job can be traced back to the ups and downs of self-esteem when individuals with fragile selfs try to use others to make themselves feel stronger and more whole.
>
> (p. 42)

It is also important to keep in mind, as Stolorow (1986) noted, that selfobject failure does not refer to objectively assessed shortcomings of the other person, but rather to a "subjectively experienced absence of requisite selfobject functions" (p. 389).

One of the reasons a focus on the selfobject dimension of precipitating events is so important is for the light it sheds on the state of the self, the quality of the patient's selfobject world and the connection between the two. There is generally an inverse relationship between the strength of the internal psychic structure and the strength of the external selfobject surround. When less has been organized internally, more is needed externally. Thus, the individual is more vulnerable to disruptions in those externally stimulated selfobject experiences. Conversely, the more cohesively organized one's internal experience is, the less vulnerable the individual is to the vicissitudes of the selfobject surround or to debilitating narcissistic injury in the face of selfobject failure.

Thus, one person's wobble is another person's earthquake. One person can shrug off the boss's scowl as reflecting a bad mood, while a coworker is devastated by even a hint of criticism. This is why a knowledge of external events tells us nothing without a corresponding understanding of their meaning to the patient.

That meaning has to be understood with a great deal of specificity. For example, one patient reported that marine boot camp was one of the best periods of his life. Surprised by this statement, I encouraged him to elaborate. He described how competent he felt at doing what was required of him physically and how much he enjoyed the sameness of uniforms and haircuts. It became clear that he loved boot camp for its structure, discipline and challenge. These qualities, which had been sorely lacking in his family growing up, helped him with self-regulation, self-esteem and a sense of belonging. Conversely, when he was off the base and not in uniform, his military haircut made him feel painfully *out* of place and contributed to a discomfort which ultimately was so intolerable he decided to leave the service.

Basch (1992, 1995) constantly enjoined therapists to get examples when a patient described a problem, believing that it was the specific details which would clarify the meaning of the events and issues the patient reported.

When someone reports difficulty getting over a relationship, I've found it particularly helpful to ask, "What do you think about when you think about him (or her)?" Does the person describe missing the affirmation of an admirer, the company of a playmate or the solace of being held in the dark of the night? These point to differing internal experiences and needs.

In describing her boyfriend, one patient said, "Don is amazing ... when he holds me his strength just seems to flow into me, wrapping around me and keeping me safe." When she later broke up with Don, the lost selfobject experience for her was very different from the woman described earlier who struggled with her appearance after her boyfriend left.

This question of what the patient thinks about is relevant to any loss, whether of a relationship, a job, or health and faculties. It is equally relevant to new challenges. Moving away from home, starting a new school or job, getting married, having a baby and retiring are all life changes that have highly subjective, personal meanings.

For one patient, struggling with feelings of depletion after leaving her large and chaotic family, the significance of the change was in the loss of stimulation provided by all the commotion and activity at home. Suddenly on her own, her underlying emptiness became apparent. The appropriate focus of treatment was not anxiety about either separation or the new challenges she faced, but rather the need for external stimulation in order to mobilize or sustain any sense of vitality.

For another woman, who spent years nursing a failing spouse, her husband's death triggered a loss of structure and meaning. Her sense of self had become organized around the caregiving role, a pattern not uncommon for people in her situation. Treating this only as a problem of grief and mourning would miss what in fact became a more relevant concern for the treatment: finding a new basis for a sense of purpose, in order to restore her self-esteem. Finding new ways to sustain self-esteem constitutes a very different focus for treatment than resolution of an object loss or grief reaction.

Sometimes what is lost is a hope or fantasy. Bergart (1997) studied the losses and challenges involved when a woman closes the door on unsuccessful fertility treatment. Both Moses (1987) and Fajardo (1987) described the loss of dreams when a parent gives birth to a disabled child. Benetar (1989) similarly outlined the narcissistic issues stimulated in parents when their children marry someone very different from the parents' wishes and expectations.

The question of what comes to mind when the patient thinks about the presenting problem is helpful when dealing with trauma as well as loss. The specifics of traumatic memories provide clues to the nature of the underlying problem, continuing difficulties or both. This is true of a wide range of situations, including assaults, accidents and abuse.

When a hospital chaplain told me she was stymied by a patient who seemed unable to resolve the death of his wife, I asked her what he talked about when he talked about his spouse. In fact, the man always returned to exactly the same point, the experience of discovering her in the bathroom, dead of cardiac arrest, shortly after bringing her home from the hospital. Rather than suffering from an unresolved grief reaction, he was suffering from an acute anxiety reaction, more specifically post-traumatic stress, triggered by the way in which he discovered his wife's death. What he needed was help in integrating the shock, the sense of helplessness and the other affects connected with this traumatic memory. This is, again, a very different focus from his grief over his lost partner.

This example, as well as several of the ones above, brings to mind what I consider the quintessential story for brief treatment.[4] As the story goes, an army general, very frustrated when his men are unable to fix his broken jeep in a foreign land, calls for a local mechanic. After looking under the hood for a bit, the mechanic asks for a hammer and gives the engine a bang. To the general's amazement, the car starts right up. Impressed and grateful, the happy general asks how much he owes. The mechanic says, "That will be $100." Taken aback, the general responds, "$100? For one bang?" "No," said the mechanic. "$1 for the bang, and $99 for knowing *where* to bang."

For treatment to be brief, we need to avoid wasting time either trying to address the wrong problem or trying to solve a problem on the wrong level. Using an empathic mode of observation to investigate the patient's subjective experience of precipitating events and problems helps us know "where to bang," where the internal problem in the self is.

As described earlier, ultimately our inquiry always comes back to understanding the ways in which the self is vulnerable or disrupted and to establishing a selfobject relationship which will strengthen vitality and cohesion. The more rapidly we can translate the precipitants, symptoms, deficits, strengths and transferences into statements about the organization of self experience, the more readily we will be able to do this.

It is through an empathic mode of observation, facilitated by the questions described above, that we are able to understand the selfobject dimension and subjective meaning of the patient's experience. It is through empathic interpretations that we communicate that understanding to the patient.

Addressing Selfobject Experience Through Empathic Interpretations

Empathic interpretations accept, understand and explain the meaning of the patient's experiences (A. Ornstein, 1986), including their frustrated selfobject needs or longings. Understanding phenomena from the point of view of the patient's subjective experience allows the therapist to offer the selfobject responsiveness needed to restore cohesion and enable symptoms to abate.

To illustrate, using an empathic interpretation to capture his patient's experience of losing his girlfriend, one therapist declared, "When she left it was like all your good feelings about yourself walked out with her." Another therapist, responding to a young man who was upset by the cold water his father had thrown on his ideas, replied, "You wanted support for your plan and an expression of confidence in you, not twenty questions about how you'd get it to work." When the patient's older brother offered a similarly disappointing response to an accomplishment, the therapist said, "You wanted him to take pride and pleasure in your achievement, not be competitive and resentful about it."

Such interpretations belatedly legitimize underlying needs or wishes. We are accustomed to reflecting the feelings which are reactive to needs not getting met, usually feelings of hurt, anger, sadness or disappointment. But when we go beyond these reactive affects to the underlying longings and fantasies, our interpretations can have a powerful mutative effect. As Goldberg (1973) observed:

> Behind the sadness of the adolescent who is rejected for a date is the image of a dashing and irresistible hero whom no one can resist. His anger at the girl who turns him down is secondary to feeling injured. Relief comes when someone can understand the hidden image of himself without ridicule or condemnation. Behind the disabling depression of the chronically ill is the fantasy of the perfect body that is intact and beautiful and cannot be damaged.
>
> (p. 726)

A cancer patient, successfully treated in brief psychotherapy for problems stimulated by her illness, described feeling enraged when people told her that the way she felt was "normal" when it was anything but normal for her. What she wanted was understanding, not reassurance that couldn't really be offered. When the doors closed behind the people leaving the room where she received radiation, she wanted someone to simply appreciate the fear she felt at that moment, to understand her sense of aloneness and helplessness. She needed this experience accepted and confirmed.

An elderly man home alone recovering from major surgery complained that the physical therapist wasn't showing up and his home-delivered meals weren't coming on time. Looking at the internal meaning of his situation, it becomes clearer that he was upset at being failed by those who were supposed to take care of him, adding salt to the injury that he couldn't take care of himself. He missed his strong, capable body and was disappointed and furious with the idealized caregivers who were not coming through for him.

He railed at the therapist, "I'm still waiting for my meals, can you believe it? I am so upset, I don't know what to do! I can't get well. I want to get strong, so I can go out. Do you understand?!" She replied, "I do. I understand that you are trying to get better, stronger, how you used to be. You want to recover from the surgery, so that you can get back to doing all these things like cooking meals for yourself, so you won't have to wait for a delivery. And the fact that you have to wait, sometimes not getting meals, is standing right in the way of your getting better, getting back to where you want to be. It's frustrating you in reaching your goal." With a huge sigh and great sense of relief, he replied, "Yes, exactly, that's it." He wanted her to appreciate his destination, not just his frustration.

The use of empathic interpretations to clarify and legitimize needs, affect and experience is a crucial mutative tool in any self psychologically informed treatment. In brief treatment, it occupies center stage. We constantly articulate our understanding of what events and experiences mean to the patient, and we do so in a very active, explicit and ongoing way.

In addition to its general mutative power, using an empathic mode of observation and response to focus on internal experience and specific meanings also saves time because of its power to mitigate defensiveness and resistance. Consider, for example, this excerpt from the second session of a brief treatment case:

PT: I don't understand why I am here with you, you're just going to send me home after we talk. Maybe I should leave now.

TH: You're worried that what we do here won't be enough. You're wondering if it's even worth it.

PT: Sometimes I think I'd be better off in the hospital for a while. Then I could try to deal with everything that has happened to me. I wouldn't have to worry about being strong and responsible or taking care of everyone else.

TH: Although you're feeling a lot of your own pain, you don't feel you have time to deal with that because you're too busy taking care of everyone else. Perhaps you see the hospital as a place where you'd have permission to stop worrying about everyone else and just take care of *you* for a while.

PT: Yes. Even when I'm here with you, I'm thinking about everything else I have to do. I can't let myself focus on all my problems, or let you push me to talk about them, because when I go home I have to be strong and pretend like everything is okay. No one would know what to do if *I* fell apart. Who would take care of me?

TH: You want to know that someone cares about you and would take care of you if *you* fell apart.

PT: You don't care about me. You're only here because it's your job, picking people apart! You're supposed to open me up so you can see what's wrong with me, explain it to me, and then leave me to deal with it. You know, just when the going gets tough, you get going!

TH: So you expect that I'll open you up and then just leave you all alone to deal with what's wrong, right when you most need my help. From what you said earlier, this is something you have experienced before. You've gotten used to people getting inside you and then rejecting what they see. You're afraid that I will do the same thing, and you don't want to be hurt like that again.

At this point the patient began to cry. The therapist's empathic attunement and understanding, of both her wishes and her fears (i.e., the protective functions of her anger and defensiveness), enabled her to feel understood. Her affect changed markedly as she began to talk about her earlier experiences of rejection, expressing painful feelings in a way she had previously been unable to do.

In describing the profound effect on the state of the self which this kind of empathic understanding has, P. Ornstein and A. Ornstein (1996) explained, "Feeling understood is the adult equivalent of being held, which on the level of self-experience results in firming up or consolidating the self" (p. 94). The underlying feelings and needs made available by the ensuing suspension of defense are then integrated and transformed through the therapist's empathic interpretations.

In the example above, the therapist sought to convey her understanding without further investigation of her own contribution, in the present, to the patient's experience of the therapist as someone who didn't care about her, wanted to push her to talk, would pick her apart and would leave her to deal with her problems alone. This would be an appropriate and expected focus in a self psychologically informed treatment and certainly could have been meaningfully pursued here. At the same time, it is important for the brief therapist to realize that an empathic interpretation of the patient's subjective experience, without such exploration of the joint contributions of both parties to that experience, may be sufficient to mitigate defensiveness and gain access to underlying affects.

To summarize, empathic interpretations constitute the therapist's most powerful tool for communicating understanding, clarifying experience, legitimizing affect and needs, mitigating defensiveness, facilitating the reorganization of affective experience and strengthening the self. In addition, for most patients the experience of being responded to in this way constitutes a new relational experience, which is in itself a potent aspect of the mutative process.

Addressing Something without Addressing Everything

Correction in Course

With brief treatment, our goal is less to get something finished than to get something started. We're aiming for a correction in course. Whether what gets started is a process of understanding, of stabilization or of change, we're trying to strengthen the self, to help the patient develop more internal and external resources for dealing with life. This process does not need to be completed at the time of termination for continued working through and growth to occur afterwards.[5]

In other words, in brief treatment, we can address *something* without addressing *everything*. Yet a little bit can go a long way. Sometimes what the patient emerges with is a new experience of what is possible, both in relation to themselves and to others. One patient, faced with the need to end treatment because her therapist was moving away, said, "All my life I was waiting for someone who could understand me. You came along and now you're leaving and I won't have that anymore." After reflecting the patient's feelings of loss, the therapist added, "So you'll never again have the experience of feeling that there's no one who could ever understand you." "Right," the patient responded, "it makes me feel like less of a freak."

The therapist's response to this isolated and disconnected woman underscored that there was some experience of the relationship that would remain with her, whatever else might be lost in their termination. Once she has felt understood in this way, she can no longer go back to seeing herself as incomprehensible or the world as a place where such an empathic connection would never be possible. She might believe that it will never happen again. However, much as the task of clearing a path in the woods which has become overgrown is much less difficult than the task of carving it out the first time, finding one's way back to an experience is usually easier than getting there initially. This patient's experience with her therapist opens the door to her being able to seek out and find similar experiences with others.

Mutative Moments

Experiences like those of the woman just described are powerful events which can permanently change the internal landscape. Elson (1995), encouraging therapists doing brief treatment to appreciate the enormous potential of even brief encounters, drew on an experience of Dostoevsky's to illustrate:

> We not infrequently despair over the brevity of our work with the individuals who come to us or are mandated for treatment. I would like to share an illustration of the manner in which a weakened and endangered self can be sustained by the brief experience of a selfobject function which becomes transformed into psychic structure capable of restoring cohesion and strength to that self.
>
> When Dostoevsky was but twenty four, he spent more than a year revising and editing a work of fiction called *Poor Folk*. Finally he read it to a friend, who in turn showed it to other friends, who woke him in the middle of the night to give him hugs and congratulations. One friend took it to a much feared and revered Russian critic, urging him to read the manuscript and likening its author to a new Gogol. Skeptical at first, he roared, "Bring him to me!" His enthusiasm and praise were unstinting. And Dostoevsky left him in a daze, wondering, "Am I really such a great man?"
>
> Many years later he wrote, "This was the most blissful moment of my life. Every time I remembered this moment when I was in Siberia

(where his wrists and ankles were shackled for four years, leaving permanent scars) I found new courage and strength. Still today I remember it with joy."

(Geir Kjetsa, Fyodor Dostoevsky:
A Writer's Life, 1987, p. 45).

Our clients and patients perhaps do not have the genius of a Dostoevsky, yet the experience of being the center and focus of our empathic attention, the experience of being understood, does not go away. It remains as a beacon and may assist an individual in his lifelong quest for meaningful goals and relationships.

As therapists, we can reflect on moments both in our own lives and in our own treatment when this kind of powerful experience left a lasting impression. We might think of our appreciation of small gestures of understanding when grief stricken, our swelling with pride when affirmed by someone we particularly admire or our deep sense of connection and well being when someone responds to us by sharing their own experience in a way which makes us feel known and understood in the depth of our being. It is not the duration, but the affective intensity of such experiences, which gives them their tremendous mutative power.

Termination: Object Loss and Selfobject Loss

When termination occurs before the therapist or patient feels the work is fully done, which is often the case in brief treatment, there can be concern about what will be lost by stopping. It is helpful here to distinguish between object loss, which concerns the therapist as a separate, valued person who might be missed or mourned, and selfobject loss, which has to do with sustaining functions or experiences of which the therapist has been the source. When selfobject loss is a concern, there is a fear that with the loss of the therapist will come a loss, for example, of the capacity to be self-regulating, the ability to calm or motivate oneself or (like the patient above) the opportunity to be understood and appreciated. One patient, preparing to end his brief psychotherapy, asked the therapist for a tangible possession, something of hers that would be a reminder (or transitional object) to aid in his struggle to internalize their bond and the functions it provided (Gardner, 1991).

When we evaluate how people might do after termination, this selfobject dimension of the relationship is important to examine. It is helpful to ask ourselves what the patient will be able to sustain internally without us, either because there has been an increase in self-esteem or self-regulating capacities and the self is more firmly structured, or because there has been an expansion of the selfobject milieu and the person is better able to find others who can be a source of sustaining selfobject experiences. These are connected; one has to believe a feeling or need is legitimate before one dares to express or seek to meet it. Being validated in therapy leads to more ability to assert one's needs outside of therapy.

It is useful to talk to people directly about these issues. One patient, announcing she no longer felt the need for me, stated, "I can validate myself now." Some people have described how they imagined writing in a journal or turning more to other people to sort out their feelings, once they stopped coming to therapy. Others described recalling specific words I'd said or concepts we'd discussed, to help them stay calm or hopeful when anxiety or despair threatened to overwhelm them.

Keeping in mind that brief treatment often ends at a time when the structure-building process and reorganization of self experience have been set in motion but not completed, it is appropriate to help patients think through the consequences of leaving the selfobject matrix of the therapy relationship. This can best be accomplished by exploring together the current state of the patient's internal and external resources for sustaining a cohesive and vital sense of self.

Components of a Model to Facilitate Briefer Treatment

Earlier I stated that the model I describe is less a particular technique than a series of components, whose combined use can make treatment more efficient. These components include:

1. Eliciting patient expectations and active collaboration in defining the goals of treatment, reinforcing the patient as a center of initiative in the process;
2. Emphasizing and using the patient's strengths;
3. Illuminating and addressing underlying vulnerabilities which are exposed when usual defenses and solutions are overwhelmed;

4. Using an empathic mode of observation to focus on the selfobject dimension (internal meaning) of precipitating events; and
5. Using empathic interpretations to clarify and validate subjective experience, needs and frustrated longings.

There is nothing new in these activities *per se* or different from what one might do in long-term treatment. But any one of them might be less emphasized in longer term therapy. That is not the case here. It is the combined and active use of *all* of these steps which makes the difference.

Focus is crucial, in both assessment and intervention. We are constantly looking for specific things, through particular lenses. We look, for example, not simply at precipitating events, but at the selfobject dimension of those events. By utilizing strengths and clarifying vulnerabilities, we can move rapidly to the interpretation of focal issues.

Careful assessment of changes in the state of the self and associated selfobject surround, using the frameworks described above, to determine how self experience is vulnerable to disruption enables the therapist to understand what must be addressed in order to enhance the self's vitality and cohesion. When we then communicate our understanding of the patient's subjective experience through empathic interpretations, we strengthen the self, mitigate defensiveness, facilitate the formation of a selfobject bond and provide a new relational experience, all of which advance the therapeutic process.

Once this process has been mobilized, it may well continue on its own momentum after the treatment relationship ends. Thus, a correction in course, rather than a completed journey, may be sufficient to produce benefit from brief treatment.[5]

Although developed in the context of long-term, intensive psychotherapy and psychoanalysis, the conceptual framework provided by self psychology is ideally suited to facilitate treatment of any duration, no matter how brief. When translated from theory to practice, this framework provides a roadmap which can help us use whatever time we have to maximally help our patients.

Notes

1 Those seeking a comprehensive overview of contemporary self psychology are also referred to the excellent summary statement provided by Fosshage (1998).
2 In his final book, Basch (1995) actually dropped the term "idealization" and began using the word "reliance" to denote this aspect of the patient's needs and transference.

3 For sake of convenience, I use the term "the self" in the remainder of this chapter to refer to the subjective sense of self and to the organization of self experience. I do not mean to imply, by this term, an entity, agent or fixed structure.
4 I don't know who originated this story, but credit Leo Bellak with bringing it into the domain of brief dynamic treatment.
5 For a detailed clinical report of changes that were achieved and those still in progress at the time of termination in brief treatment, see chapter 3 in this volume.

References

Bacal, H. (1985). Optimal responsiveness and the therapeutic process. In A. Goldberg (Ed.), *Progress in self psychology, Vol. I* (pp. 202–227). New York, NY: Guilford.

Bacal, H. (1990). The elements of a corrective selfobject experience. *Psychoanalytic Inquiry, 10,* 347–372.

Bacal, H. (1998). *Optimal responsiveness: How therapists heal their patients.* Northvale, NJ: Jason Aronson.

Baker, H. (1991). Shorter-term psychotherapy: A self psychological approach. In P. Crits-Christoph & J. Barber (Eds.), *Handbook of short-term dynamic psychotherapy* (pp. 287–322). New York, NY: Basic Books.

Balint, M., Ornstein, P., & Balint, E. (1972). *Focal psychotherapy: An example of applied psychoanalysis.* London, UK: Tavistock.

Basch, M.F. (1980). *Doing psychotherapy.* New York, NY: Basic Books.

Basch, M.F. (1988). *Understanding psychotherapy: The science behind the art.* New York, NY: Basic Books.

Basch, M.F. (1992). *Practicing psychotherapy: A casebook.* New York, NY: Basic Books.

Basch, M.F. (1995). *Doing brief psychotherapy.* New York, NY: Basic Books.

Beebe, B., & Lachmann, F. (1988). Mother-infant mutual influence and precursors of psychic structure. In *Progress in self psychology, volume 3* (pp. 3–26). Hillsdale, NJ: Analytic Press.

Bellak, L., & Small, L. (1978). *Emergency psychotherapy and brief psychotherapy* (2nd ed.). New York, NY: Grune & Stratton.

Benetar, M. (1989). "Marrying off" children as a developmental stage. *Clinical Social Work Journal, 17,* 223–231.

Bergart, A. (1997). *Women's views of their lives after infertility treatment fails* (Unpublished doctoral dissertation). University of Chicago.

Chernus, L. (1983). Focal psychotherapy and self pathology: A clinical illustration. *Clinical Social Work Journal, 11,* 215–227.

Elson, M. (1986). *Self psychology in clinical social work.* New York, NY: Norton.

Elson, M. (1989). Kohut and Stern: Two views of infancy and early childhood. *Smith College Studies in Social Work, 59,* 131–145.

Elson, M. (1995, April). *Pathways to health in self psychology.* Paper presented at the Seventy Second Annual Meeting, American Orthopsychiatric Association, Chicago, IL.

Fajardo, B. (1987). Parenting a damaged child: Mourning, regression, and disappointment. *Psychoanalytic Review, 74,* 19–43.

Fosshage, J. (1998). Self psychology and its contributions to psychoanalysis: An overview. *Journal of Analytic Social Work, 5,* 1–17.

Gardner, J. (1991). The application of self psychology to brief psychotherapy. *Psychoanalytic Psychology, 8,* 477–500.

Gardner, J. (1999). Using self psychology in brief psychotherapy. *Psychoanalytic Social Work, 6,* 43–85.

Goldberg, A. (1973). Psychotherapy of narcissistic injuries. *Archives of General Psychiatry, 28,* 722–726.

Kohut, H. (1959). Introspection, empathy and psychoanalysis. *Journal of the American Psychoanalytic Association, 7,* 459–483.

Kohut, H. (1966). Forms and transformations of narcissism. *Journal of the American Psychoanalytic Association, 14,* 243–272.

Kohut, H. (1971). *The analysis of the self.* New York, NY: International Universities Press.

Kohut, H. (1977). *The restoration of the self.* New York, NY: International Universities Press.

Kohut, H. (1984). *How does analysis cure?* Chicago, IL: University of Chicago Press.

Kohut, H. (1987). *The Kohut seminars on self psychology and psychotherapy with adolescents and young adults* (M. Elson, Ed.). New York, NY: Norton.

Kohut, H. (1996). *The Chicago Institute Lectures* (P. Tolpin & M. Tolpin, Eds.). Hillsdale, NJ: The Analytic Press.

Kohut, H., & Wolf, E.S. (1978). Disorders of the self and their treatment. *International Journal of Psychoanalysis, 59,* 413–425.

Lazarus, L. (1980). Brief psychotherapy of narcissistic disturbances. *Psychotherapy: Theory, Research and Practice, 19,* 228–236.

Lazarus, L. (1988). Self psychology: Its application to brief psychotherapy with the elderly. *Journal of Geriatric Psychiatry, 21,* 109–125.

Lichtenberg, J. (1989). *Psychoanalysis and motivation.* Hillsdale, NJ: Analytic Press.

Lichtenberg, J. (1991). What is a selfobject? *Psychoanalytic Dialogues, 1,* 455–479.

Lichtenberg, J., Lachmann, F., & Fosshage, J. (1992). *Self and motivational systems: Toward a theory of technique.* Hillsdale, NJ: Analytic Press.

Lichtenberg, J., Lachmann, F., & Fosshage, J. (1996). *The clinical exchange: Technique derived from self and motivational systems.* Hillsdale, NJ: Analytic Press.

Messer, S., & Warren, C. (1995). *Models of brief psychodynamic therapy: A comparative approach.* New York, NY: The Guilford Press.

Moses, K. (1987). The impact of childhood disability: The parent's struggle. *Ways, 6,* 6–10.

Orange, D. (1995). *Emotional understanding: Studies in psychoanalytic epistemology.* New York, NY: The Guilford Press.

Ornstein, A. (1986). "Supportive" psychotherapy: A contemporary view. *Clinical Social Work Journal, 14,* 14–30.

Ornstein, A., & Ornstein, P. (1986). Empathy and the therapeutic dialogue. In *The Lydia Rappaport lecture series* (pp. 3–16). Northampton, MA: Smith School of Social Work.

Ornstein, A., & Ornstein, P. (1996). II. Speaking in the interpretive mode and feeling understood: Crucial aspects of the therapeutic action in psychotherapy. In L. Lifson (Ed.), *Understanding therapeutic action: Psychodynamic concepts of cure* (pp. 103–125). Hillsdale, NJ: The Analytic Press.

Ornstein, A., & Ornstein, P. (1997, November). *Brief but deep: Finding the focus in "focal psychotherapy."* Paper presented at the Twentieth Annual International Conference on the Psychology of the Self, Chicago, IL.

Ornstein, P. (1988). Multiple curative factors and processes in the psychoanalytic psychotherapies. In A. Rothstein (Ed.), *How does treatment help?* (Workshop Series of the American Psychoanalytic Association, Monograph 4, pp. 105–126). Madison, CT: International Universities Press.

Ornstein, P., & Ornstein, A. (1972). Focal psychotherapy: Its potential impact on psychotherapeutic practice in medicine. *Journal of Psychiatry in Medicine, 3*, 311–325.

Ornstein, P., & Ornstein, A. (1977). On the continuing evolution of psychoanalytic psychotherapy: Reflections and predictions. *The Annual of Psychoanalysis, 5*, 329–370.

Ornstein, P., & Ornstein, A. (1996). I. Some general principles of psychoanalytic psychotherapy: A self-psychological perspective. In L. Lifson (Ed.), *Understanding therapeutic action: Psychodynamic concepts of cure* (pp. 87–101). Hillsdale, NJ: The Analytic Press.

Ringstrom, P. (1995). Exploring the model scene: Finding the focus in an intersubjective approach to brief psychotherapy. *Psychoanalytic Inquiry, 15*, 493–513.

Seruya, B. (1997). *Empathic brief psychotherapy*. Northvale, NJ: Jason Aronson.

Shane, M., Shane, E., & Gales, M. (1997). *Intimate attachments: Towards a new self psychology*. New York: The Guilford Press.

Socarides, D., & Stolorow, R. (1984–1985). Affects and selfobjects. *The Annual of Psychoanalysis, 12/13*, 105–119.

Stolorow, R. (1986). Critical reflections on the theory of self psychology: An inside view. *Psychoanalytic Inquiry, 6*, 387–402.

Stolorow, R. (1998). Foreword. In I. Hardwood & M. Pines (Eds.), *Self experiences in group: Intersubjective and self psychological pathways to human understanding* (pp. 7–8). London, UK: Jessica Kingsley Publishers.

Stolorow, R., & Atwood, G. (1992). *Contexts of being: The intersubjective foundations of psychological life*. Hillsdale, NJ: The Analytic Press.

Stolorow, R., Brandchaft, B., & Atwood, G. (1987). *Psychoanalytic treatment: An intersubjective approach*. Hillsdale, NJ: The Analytic Press.

Terman, D. (1988). Optimum frustration: Structuralization and the therapeutic process. In A. Goldberg (Ed.), *Learning from Kohut: Progress in self psychology, vol. 4* (pp. 113–126). Hillsdale, NJ: Analytic Press.

Terman, D. (1989). Therapeutic change: Perspectives of self psychology. *Psychoanalytic Inquiry, 9*, 88–100.

Tolpin, M. (1971). On the beginnings of a cohesive self. *The Psychoanalytic Study of the Child, 26*, 316–352.

Tolpin, M. (1983). Corrective emotional experience: A self psychological reevaluation. In A. Goldberg (Ed.), *The future of psychoanalysis* (pp. 363–380). New York, NY: International Universities Press.

Tolpin, M., & Kohut, H. (1980). The disorders of the self: The psychopathology of the first years of life. In S.I. Greenspan & G.H. Pollock (Eds.), *The course of life* (pp. 425–442). Bethesda, MD: NIMH.

Tolpin, P. (1984). Discussion of "A current perspective on difficult patients" by B. Brandchaft and R. D. Stolorow, and "Issues in the treatment of the borderline patient" by G. Adler. In A. Goldberg & P. Stepansky (Eds.), *Kohut's legacy* (pp. 138–142). Hillsdale, NJ: Analytic Press.

Wolf, E.S. (1980). On the developmental line of selfobject relations. In A. Goldberg (Ed.), *Advances in self psychology* (pp. 117–130). New York, NY: International Universities Press.

Wolf, E.S. (1988). *Treating the self: Elements of clinical self psychology*. New York, NY: Guilford.

Chapter 4

Supervision of Trainees

Continuing the efforts to extend and apply self psychological theory beyond the practice of psychoanalysis, this chapter examines how self psychology can be useful in the process of training psychotherapists in a variety of clinical and community settings. Clinical supervision is seen here as instrumental in the development, consolidation and mainte-nance of a cohesive professional self. By establishing a selfobject bond in which the anxieties and vulnerabilities of the trainee can be managed, the supervisor facilitates the maintenance of self-esteem and expansion of cognitive understanding. Accomplishing these aims involves form-ing an empathic alliance with the internal, subjective experience of the supervisee. How to focus on the therapist-in-training's selfobject needs via an empathic mode of observation and response is illustrated by sev-eral examples and vignettes, chosen from a variety of clinical settings and modalities of treatment. As in the previous chapters, this one empha-sizes the blending of theoretical concepts with practical concerns and applications.

This paper was published in 1995 as "Supervision of Trainees: Tending the Professional Self" in the Clinical Social Work Journal, *Volume 23.*

Professionals often "graduate" to supervisory roles with little or no for-mal training in how to conceptualize the supervisory process. In this chapter, I approach clinical supervision of therapists in training as an activity which includes among its fundamental aims the development, consolidation and maintenance of a cohesive professional self. The term "professional" self is used here to refer to those aspects of self structure and experience which come into play when one is functioning in one's chosen, vocational arena.

DOI: 10.4324/9781003491453-5

Selfobject Experience in the Supervisory Relationship

Theorists in self psychology conceptualize psychotherapy as a structure-building process which has as its central goal the strengthening of the self (Kohut, 1977, 1984; Wolf, 1988). An emphasis on the self experience of the patient and the selfobject dimension (Stolorow, 1986) of the therapeutic relationship is at the heart of self psychological thinking.

The concepts of selfobject experience, needs, transference and counter-transference are equally relevant to the supervisory relationship, which is also a structure-building process in which selfobject needs are expressed, and to various degrees met, by both parties. Supervisor and supervisee form a self-selfobject unit, through which the trainee's anxieties and vulnerabilities can be managed in the service of consolidating a cohesive professional self.

Elson (1989) has described the selfobject dimension this way:

> To undertake new learning exposes individuals to anxiety that they may not succeed, that failure and shame may be the outcome. The adult learner experiences the arousal of feelings of earliest pleasurable expectation but also of helplessness, of the need to have a meaningful image of himself mirrored, confirmed, and guided, and of the need to merge with the strength and wisdom of an idealized selfobject.
>
> (p. 796)

Muslin and Val (1989) also described learning as requiring specific selfobject functions for self-esteem regulation. However, they saw individuals as differing in the timing, nature and form that these needs take. This leads to a need for the supervisor to make an "empathic diagnosis of the learner's selfobject needs" (p. 161) at any given point in the student's development. While they described the self-sustaining functions of mirroring as crucial for some people, they observed that learning can and does also occur without echoing and confirming attitudes from the supervisor. Similarly, the extent of idealization varies: "some teachers are experienced as messianic figures who speak with omniscience while others are experienced as partners who offer suggestions" (p. 162). These different profiles are seen as reflecting both the extent to which the learner needs to idealize and the extent to which the supervisor is comfortable in accepting the idealization.

An unpublished paper by Reams suggests a developmental progression or sequence of selfobject needs in supervision. The beginning student, feeling overwhelmed, may be more likely to seek idealized selfobjects who can provide strength and structure. As the student begins to gain in strength and have more autonomous ideas, there is an increased need for an audience to mirror the student's efforts and emerging professional self. As supervisees start to feel more like competent professionals on their own, they may wish to validate their entry into the membership of accomplished therapists by joining in a sense of twinship with the supervisor. Friedman and Kaslow (1986) described a similar progression in students' needs for varying kinds of supervisory support and response over the course of training.

In a paper outlining the development of professional self-concepts, Brightman (1984) detailed the narcissistic vulnerability of the therapist in training. He describes student aspirations as initially reflecting a triad of idealized attributes which determine professional self-esteem: omniscience, benevolence and omnipotence. Together, they comprise the student's "grandiose professional self," an image of oneself as the all-knowing, all-loving, all-powerful therapist. Trainees' actual clinical experiences quickly confront them with the unrealistic aspects of this image, and, as the real and idealized versions of their professional self-image inevitably collide, they face the threat of narcissistic injury and a precipitous loss of self-esteem.

To manage the tension generated by this struggle between the demands of clinical training, their novice level of skill and their perfectionistic aspirations, Brightman explained, students need and seek the support of an understanding, caring and competent supervisor. A relationship with such an idealized mentor provides a holding environment (Winnicott, 1965) in which the "grandiose" professional self-image can be modified toward a more moderate and attainable ego-ideal. As the trainee's belief in his or her professional worth grows, the need to be part of someone else's competence diminishes and a gradual de-idealization process occurs.

The student therapist's selfobject needs are expressed not only in the relationship with the supervisor, but also in the relationship with the patient. Several people have written about the normal, non-pathological need for the patient to function as a confirming selfobject for the therapist's professional self (Adler, 1984; Bacal, 1992; Barth, 1988; Wolf, 1983). The patient's actual behavior may serve to meet, overstimulate or frustrate the therapist's selfobject needs (Wolf, 1983). For example, the patient's idealization may be uncomfortably stimulating to the therapist's grandiosity, while the patient's depreciation may be painfully wounding to it. Many negative countertransference reactions stem from the lack of validation for his or her professional competence that the therapist feels when he cannot soothe or hold the patient, i.e., when the therapist has an experience of failure or rejection as an adequate selfobject for the patient (Adler, 1984). In the early stages of training, much supervisory attention must be devoted to helping students deal with these frustrated needs for validation and efficacy.

The supervisor's selfobject needs are also mobilized in the teaching and learning process of supervision, and, like the trainee's, these needs are to varying degrees either met or frustrated by the supervisory experience. Although the supervisor's professional self-esteem is generally much less vulnerable than that of the neophyte, it, too, is sustained by experiences of idealization and affirming responsiveness. Frustration of the supervisor's need to be proud of his or her "professional progeny" or to receive grateful affirmation of the supervisor's helpfulness and knowledge can lead to supervisory countertransference enactments which reflect the supervisor's own feelings of incompetence, failure and lowered self-esteem. Awareness and understanding of these feelings are crucial if the supervisor is to sustain the requisite selfobject matrix for the trainee.

Another dimension of countertransference experience to which both supervisor and supervisee need to stay finely attuned has to do with the process of affective resonance or attunement. This is the process by which the feeling states aroused in the therapist provide valuable clues to the patient's internal state. Beginning therapists often feel ashamed of their negative feelings and try to disavow them, not realizing that these feelings can be used diagnostically as legitimate and valuable sources of information about the self states of their patients.

A student therapist described to her supervisor feelings of helplessness and withdrawal from her patient, a sense that she had nothing to say to the patient. The therapist was apologetic about these feelings, which she took as a sign of failure on her part. She felt unable to grasp the patient's experience in any useful way. And yet, after a brief period of supervisory dialogue, it became quite clear that a similar sense of helplessness was at the crux of the patient's current feelings, as well as a feeling in the patient that her only viable response was to withdraw into passivity. The supervisor helped the therapist realize that rather than criticizing herself for her feelings, she could use them to understand her patient.

In another example, a therapist came into supervision wondering how to interpret or confront a patient's behavior in the milieu program where he worked. The patient was engaging in a kind of social sadism in which she would zero in on the staff's shortcomings and then make people feel extremely uncomfortable by commenting on their flaws in some disarming and embarrassing way. This left the staff feeling hostile, wary, and critical toward the patient, as well as bad about themselves. Myriad other examples of the patient's underlying low self-esteem, extreme sensitivity to injury and slights, and vulnerability to criticism suggested that these attacks on others reflected an attempt to stabilize her own shaky self-esteem, by putting others down, as well as a way to communicate something about her own inner experience. Her behavior was making the staff feel the way she felt, depreciated and worthless. Understanding the patient not as simply a hostile person venting her aggression on them, but as someone who was feeling on the inside the way she was causing them to feel, put the staff in a very different position to use those feelings, first to understand the patient and then to convey that understanding to her in some empathic way. With this shift on the part of the therapist, the patient's attacking behavior dropped markedly, and she began to talk more meaningfully about her own painful feelings.

The parallel between the patient's experience and therapist's experience of the patient, as well as its diagnostic use, also extends to the relationship with the supervisor. Gediman and Wolkenfeld (1980) describe how therapists enact patterns and processes with their supervisor which parallel those occurring in their interactions with the patient. By virtue of this parallel process, the supervisor's emotional reactions to the supervisee may shed light on what it's like for the therapist to be with the patient. For example, they cite a student who garbles his presentation so much that his supervisor can't respond in any coherent way and who then complains to the supervisor about his patient's "exasperating inarticulateness." Gediman and Wolkenfeld see this kind of countertransference as a supervisory asset: "It is as if the therapist were saying to the supervisor, 'I cannot tell you in words what the patient is like, but I can show you and make you feel what the patient is like'" (p. 239).

The everyday experience of supervisors is filled with examples of such parallel processes. Feelings of having to be very careful with a student, for instance, may reflect the therapist's similar experience with the patient. Other common examples include the supervisor's feeling helpless, attacked, confused, inundated with demands for advice and direction or frustrated because it seems that anything he or she offers is rejected. Initially, supervisors may be tempted to respond to a "yes, but..." cycle by trying to offer yet another suggestion. However, once the supervisor attends to the experience diagnostically, he or she can switch the level of the dialogue to a more relevant intervention about the process. For example, the supervisor might comment, "I'm beginning to feel that no matter what I say or suggest, it's not really going to feel very useful to you, or like it's enough. I wonder if that's how you feel with this patient sometimes." This kind of intervention opens up a new channel through which both supervisor and therapist can better understand their own and the patient's experience.

The preceding comments on countertransference underscore the fact that therapists' reactions to their patients fall into several different categories, which trainees may need help in distinguishing. Experiences of affective resonance or attunement like the ones just described can facilitate, through a process of decentering (Basch, 1988), an accurate empathic understanding of the patient's experience. These clearly differ from countertransference reactions which are primarily a function of the therapist's personal history or unresolved issues. Casement (1985) has suggested using the term "personal countertransference" for the latter and "diagnostic response" for the former. Countertransference reactions related to the frustration of the therapist's selfobject needs (Adler, 1984; Bacal, 1992; Lichtenberg, 1988; Wolf, 1983) are yet another source of the trainee's experience. Whether these include reactions to failing to meet the unrealistic expectations of the "grandiose professional self" (Brightman, 1984) or simply the lack of a sense of efficacy and value experienced when one cannot evoke a positive response from the patient, the therapist may need the attuned responsiveness of the supervisor to help manage the ensuing feelings.

I have been elaborating, to this point, the role of selfobject experience, needs, transference and countertransference in the supervisory process. As previously stated, supervisor and supervisee form a self-selfobject unit. This selfobject matrix provides for the maintenance of self-esteem and the expansion of cognitive understanding as the trainee strives to consolidate a cohesive professional self. In the next section, I will turn to the question of how this comes about. What is it that promotes the establishment of the requisite selfobject matrix? What enables structure building in the professional self to occur?

The Empathic Mode of Observation in the Supervisory Process

The method by which the goals of the supervisory process are achieved is fundamentally the same as the method by which therapists achieve their treatment goals: the unwavering use of an empathic mode of observation. It has been, from the beginning, a defining feature of self psychology to examine experience from the vantage point of the patient's subjective perspective (Kohut, 1959, 1982, 1984). The importance of focusing on subjective experience and illuminating internal reality carries over to supervision, where the supervisor has the same task in examining the therapist's work; that is, the supervisor must form an empathic alliance with the internal, subjective experience of the therapist.

The supervisor has to understand why the trainee is doing what he or she is doing (what his problem is, what her goal is) before the supervisor can help the trainee consider other ways of behaving. It is important to identify and understand the internal process within the student which led to a given intervention and to deal with that, rather than simply attending to the end product of what the student did. This involves explicating and empathizing with the therapist's dilemma. Often the student's goal or intention makes perfect sense, but the method he or she has chosen to achieve it is not effective. Having understood the therapist's underlying motives. the supervisor is then in a position to be supportive, rather than critical, about some aspect of the trainee's goal, while going on to explore better ways to accomplish it. Such a process helps protect the student's vulnerable self-esteem from injury.

Often a trainee's effort *not* to do one thing will lead either to excessive passivity or excessive activity in the session. For example, consider the following two students who were each struggling with feelings about their interpretive activity in treatment.

One trainee was extremely reluctant to make any kind of interpretation to his patients and would fall silent whenever such interventions were called for. When the supervisor commented on and inquired into this process, the trainee reported that he didn't want to "bulldoze" the patient, forcing the patient to accept truths that might not be welcome or accurate.

Rather than criticizing the student's inactivity, the supervisor readily supported his desire not to bulldoze as a reasonable and valid goal, but questioned whether it needed to be accomplished by avoiding interpretations altogether. The supervisor then offered technical assistance on such issues as the timing and phrasing of interpretations, the importance of responding empathically to patient reactions to interpretations, and so forth. By dealing with the student's underlying motivation, the supervisor could respect his need for affirmation while also helping him resolve his problem in some way other than by not making interpretations at all.

Another student seemed to be engaging in just the kind of bulldozing the first student feared. Having made an interpretation of painful affect of which the patient reported no awareness, the therapist repeatedly and adamantly insisted on the truth of her interpretation despite the patient's equally repeated and adamant denials.

Using an empathic mode of observation, the supervisor commented on the argument between patient and therapist by stating that it seemed to have been quite important to the therapist to stick to her own view of the patient's experience, despite the patient's objections. The supervisor wondered what it was that had made this goal seem so important to the therapist.

The therapist replied that she was aware of both a wish to be liked by her patient and a wish to protect the patient from the experience of painful affect, both of which she feared would be enacted by "letting the patient off the hook, not confronting her resistance, and backing off from the interpretation." In order not to yield to what she therefore perceived as inappropriate countertransference pressure to retreat, she continued to press forward with her interpretation no matter what the patient said or did.

Despite the fact that this resulted in a therapeutic impasse in which the therapist totally lost contact with her patient's experience, the supervisor was able to convey an appreciative, empathic understanding of what led the therapist into this dilemma, as well as support for the therapist's goal of basing her interventions on the patient's needs rather than her own need to be liked or to protect the patient from painful experiences. Therapist and supervisor could then embark together on an exploration of alternatives which would accomplish this goal, while also attending more effectively to the patient's needs and experience.

The supervisor's approach to the therapist's behavior in this last example is consistent with the self psychological approach to interpreting defenses and resistance (Kohut, 1984; P. Ornstein & Ornstein, 1985). The defensive behavior is not seen as something negative or dysfunctional, but rather as the individual's best available solution to protect the self from reexperiencing the trauma of injury, disappointment or empathic failure. By forming an empathic alliance with the internal, subjective experience of the trainee and understanding the adaptive functions of her behavior, rather than being critical of it, the supervisor was also offering the therapist an example and experience of this alternative approach to analyzing resistance. Needless to say, it is an approach which better safeguards the trainee's fragile self-esteem and decreases defensiveness. Because the student therapist's need for affirmation and fear of criticism are both so high, it is helpful when the supervisor responds as much as possible to what the therapist is doing right. The approach described here readily facilitates this process.

It is also important to highlight for trainees the positive aspects of their behavior because often they are engaged in a very constructive process but lack the conceptual tools to see or understand it as such. A trainee may report frustration because "nothing's happening" or complain, "I feel like I'm not doing anything if I'm just providing selfobject functions." These feelings often trigger pressured efforts to understand and explain everything on the spot or attempts to intervene quickly to relieve distress. What trainees usually need instead is a better conceptual grasp of what they are offering and how they are being used. The therapist who feels he or she is "just" providing selfobject functions, for example, generally does not understand that he or she may be offering, possibly for the first time in the patient's life, an accurately empathic and supportive selfobject milieu. Nor does the trainee recognize that the experience of this kind of responsiveness may facilitate the internalization of selfobject experiences, growth of inner psychic structure, and increased cohesion and vitality of the self. The latter includes, potentially, improvements in self-esteem, self-soothing capacities and the ability to identify and pursue ambitions and goals. Understood in this way, "just" begins to feel like quite a bit. Helping the trainee gain such conceptual understanding of his or her activities is part of the supervisor's selfobject function, by which the supervisor enables the trainee to feel engaged in a meaningful and worthwhile endeavor. It is an idealizing selfobject function of providing order and organization to experience.

Another problem for relatively new therapists is that everything the patient does seems to them to reflect something about the therapist rather than about the patient. For example, the student with a patient who is abusive, depreciating or rejecting of the therapist's help needs the support of the supervisor to understand that these behaviors say something about the patient's self experience and needs, rather than about the student's competence. The student whose new patient repeatedly cancels appointments may similarly need help in seeing that the cancellations might be reflecting the patient's ambivalence about treatment, rather than only reflecting the therapist's powers of engagement. Again, the supervisor is providing validation for the student's self-esteem, validation which is unavailable from the patient, as well as providing a cognitive framework for understanding the patient's behavior. New therapists have no way of distinguishing problems which reflect their nascent skill level from those which would occur with even the most seasoned of therapists.

Therapists in training have the additional problem of disorientation as they take in new knowledge and need help managing the feelings that accompany this. One psychology intern, for example, in the midst of learning different ways of working with people from those she had used in her previous practica, complained with despair that she felt totally at sea, not even able to remember what she used to do. She was sure it simply was all gone. The supervisor replied to her, "Just because you can't articulate your former rationale at the moment doesn't mean you don't have access to those skills, or that they aren't there and even being used. You were doing very well before you came here, in fact so well that you got into our program!" Once again, the supervisor is performing here a selfobject function of restoring continuity by reconnecting the therapist with aspects of strengths she's lost touch with.

Fuqua (1994) described this same process when she wrote about learning as a destructuring and reorganizing process. Learning involves a reorganization of what's known, which causes a disruption in self structure. According to Fuqua, the supervisor functions as a selfobject for the learner, managing these states of disruption.

The employment of empathy as a mode of observation not only helps the supervisor deal with the trainee's vulnerabilities and selfobject needs; it also directs the supervisor to the specific material which should be taken up in supervision. The trainee must be supported as a center of initiative (Kohut, 1977) in the supervisory relationship. This means focusing on the

issues and problems that the trainee finds salient and wants to resolve at any given moment.[1]

Of course, what feels most important to the therapist may not necessarily be the same as what appears most important to the supervisor. Sometimes the student therapist's technique or intervention may leave the supervisor feeling quite uneasy. Nevertheless, supervisors do best to avoid jumping in too quickly to condemn the form or content of an intervention.

There is a substantial body of literature in self psychology that underscores the idea that the manifest content of interventions may be secondary to other aspects of the therapeutic process. Stolorow's (1983) concept of "optimal empathy," Bacal's (1985) "optimal responsiveness" and P. Tolpin's (1988) "optimal affective engagement" speak to a dimension and experience of relatedness that have little to do with form or content. Terman (1988, 1989) and Miller (1991) also emphasized the central role of the selfobject bond with the therapist in promoting structure formation and a curative process. A "corrective selfobject experience" (Bacal, 1990) can take a wide variety of forms (Bacal, 1992; Gardner, 1991). A student therapist's investment in helping his or her patient may be experienced by the patient as intense interest and affirmation, even though the therapist's explanation may be in error. Kohut (1984) provided an extended example of how a Kleinian analyst making what Kohut considered a "wild" and "farfetched" interpretation nevertheless spoke to the crux of her patient's experience by conveying an accurately and warmly empathic appreciation of how distressed the patient was that the therapist had canceled one of her appointments. Similarly, a therapist's provision of direct advice and guidance at certain times might be an appropriate and optimal response to the patient's expression of idealizing needs. To criticize something a student does that is effective creates unnecessary confusion and defensiveness. We do better to keep our focus on helping the therapist realize the goals that the therapist has. It is the therapist's experience of what is not working that must be the starting point, not the supervisor's.

Of course, there are exceptions to this principle. While supervisors need a certain tolerance for less than optimal interactions by novice therapists, some issues are non-negotiable. The treatment situation must be safe, so issues involving potential harm to the patient or others, child abuse or neglect and so forth may require more initiative on the part of the supervisor. Yet this, too, is part of an effective holding environment. Just as a parent prevents a young child from running into the street,

a supervisor provides structure and direction if a trainee's patient is at serious risk or the trainee is so overwhelmed that he or she can't operate effectively. The supervisor allows the therapist to borrow the supervisor's calmness, strength and knowledge about what to do. The therapist then intervenes, experiences himself or herself as more competent and becomes less anxious. Once the situation is under control and the therapist's tension lessens, the supervisor can again invite the trainee's thoughts and speculations.

Providing more active direction to a trainee does not mean we abandon our empathic mode of observation, only that we expand it. It is always a mistake to insist in a way that isn't empathic to the therapist that a therapist be more empathic to the patient. This is like trying to treat an inadequate parent by lecturing about child rearing, an intervention which rarely helps. What does help in the parenting situation is to strengthen the parent's self so that he or she has less need to use the child to meet his or her own needs and has more to give the child. Similarly, the more the supervisor can strengthen the professional self of the therapist by understanding what the therapist is experiencing and what interferes with the therapist's being able to intervene effectively, the sooner the therapist will be able to offer the patient what he or she needs.

This is a point that is easy for supervisors to lose sight of, as illustrated in the following vignette:

A trainee with a generally cognitive/behavioral orientation to psychotherapy had approached his supervisor with an avowed interest in learning self psychology. After months of trying to help him understand how to assume a more empathic vantage point in relation to his patients' experience, the supervisor found that the student still operated largely via a highly directive, rational and educative mode of talking with them. The supervisor eventually retreated to a state of "fatigued resignation" (Brightman, 1984) in response to the therapist's ceaseless activity.

It then happened that the therapist experienced a tragedy involving a sudden death in his family and, in response to the supervisor's inquiry, spent the first supervisory meeting after his return talking entirely about this event. The supervisor listened intently during this conversation and said little, but felt intensely "with" the therapist.

Two weeks later the therapist brought a case into supervision and described how for the first time it made sense to him to just sit with his patient and listen to him: "I suddenly realized maybe I had something to offer by doing that." He then told the supervisor about his experience of their previous conversation about his family. "I never had an experience quite like that. When you spoke, I felt like your breath came through me, like you not only knew how I felt, but felt how I felt." This profound experience of empathy made a dramatic impression on him. Despite the supervisor's previous attempts to help him adopt a more empathic stance, he needed to experience it himself as something of value before he could in turn provide a similar experience to his patients.

When at the end of the year the trainee and supervisor reviewed their history together, and all their recycling in the same patterns before this breakthrough, the student asked the supervisor, "What took you so long?" After initial, failed attempts at trying to understand his experience, the supervisor had eventually met his endless harangues of his patients with harangues of her own about not making harangues.

This is reminiscent of Sloan's (1986) conclusion that trying to impart all his "pent up wisdom" about empathy to his trainees only resulted in their similarly assuming "authoritatively knowledgeable and directive roles" (p. 189) with their own patients. Sarnat (1992), too, reported stumbling on the same point:

> I realized that my own need to feel competent, interacting with [the supervisee's] characteristically passive stance, had led me to become my most dominating self. I wondered if she was perhaps providing me with an object lesson in how destructive dominating figures can be, her dictatorial tone with her patients a byproduct of the pathological interaction with me.
>
> (p. 397)

Sloan (1986) also provided a nice description of the antidote:

> The more I was able to ... acknowledge, appreciate ... or place in a larger context something of value in what my residents experienced as naturally and authentically their own (even when very different

from mine), the more confident and competent they became with their patients ... At the same time, they seemed to become more capable of adopting an empathic vantage point with their patients, which in turn brought more usable material into supervision. In short, they learned to listen best by having someone listen to them.

(p. 190)

Clinical Vignettes

The importance of attending to the self experience and selfobject needs of the therapist in training via an empathic mode of observation is illustrated in the following, more extended vignettes, which are additional examples of how the concepts I've described can be translated into practice.

Vignette #1

The patient, a young woman who had recently informed her extended family of childhood incest, had been seeking unequivocal support and validation from all family members. Any positive comments by family about the perpetrator of the abuse felt like an intolerable betrayal which canceled out their support of her.

The therapist, finding the patient's demands and expectations to be unrealistic and unreasonable, tried to confront the "splitting" that she perceived the patient to be doing. She felt the patient should take a more balanced view of how others were reacting. In response to this, the patient became more anxious and upset.

In supervision, I discussed with the therapist her patient's need to feel that the therapist was on her side. I recommended taking a more empathic position, rather than trying to help the patient perceive things more "realistically" at this point. However, as the patient continued over time to persist in these wishes for 100% agreement and support from all family members, the therapist found it difficult to be empathic to her "unrealistic demands."

Discussing the case in supervision, the therapist made it clear that she didn't experience the patient's needs as legitimate and didn't experience me as being empathic to her own experience of being with the patient. She felt that I was siding with the patient against her, with both of us accusing her of being unempathic. The therapist said that what she needed from me instead was a way to deal with, rather than discount, the feelings the patient evoked in her.

Further exploration of the therapist's experience clarified how the patient's demanding and inconsolable stance had left the therapist feeling depreciated and helpless (feelings I had been unaware of). She felt that whatever she offered was rejected and that she couldn't offer enough. The therapist sensed that I regarded these feelings as "wrong," indications that she was a bad therapist (in my eyes) and not sufficiently empathic.

In short, I had repeated with the therapist the error that was occurring in the treatment: I could only see the therapist's critical attitude toward her patients and not the inner experience behind it. I had focused continually on the legitimacy and appropriateness of the patient's inner experience and felt need for complete validation of that experience, but had not attended to what made it difficult for the therapist to experience the patient in this way.

The therapist could not make use of anything I said until she experienced her own feelings as understood by me, just as the patient could make no use of the therapist's appeals to be more "realistic" when the patient felt that her own urgent needs for validation of her traumatic experiences were not being understood or accepted by the therapist. Once I could understand the feelings of helplessness the patient evoked in the therapist, I could be more empathic to the therapist's concerns. This in turn enabled the therapist to better understand the legitimacy of her patient's experience and concerns.

Vignette #2

A marital therapist had been functioning as a sort of "switchboard" for a conflictual couple. Each partner shared complaints about the spouse with the therapist, who then responded with empathic reflections and clarifications to that individual.

I observed that while this seemed appropriate initially because of the couple's high degree of tension and misunderstanding, the treatment appeared to have progressed enough for the therapist to begin changing her role. I suggested that it might be more useful at this point for the therapist to help the couple talk directly to each other in the sessions, without the therapist acting as an intermediary.

In response to this suggestion, the therapist became aware of a strong feeling of opposition. As I encouraged her to expand on her reaction, she realized that she was reluctant to let go of her role as the understander and translator of each spouse's experience. She liked the job. She experienced the prospect of relinquishing it as a loss of a central position in these interactions, a position which made her feel competent, important and valuable in her professional role.[2]

I suggested to the therapist that she needn't be any less important in these interactions, but rather that she might be important in a different way. I suggested that the pleasure the therapist now derived from the role of being center stage in understanding her patients (the hub of the wheel) might be replaced by an equally great pleasure from witnessing her own success in facilitating an effective process of communication between two people who had previously been unable to talk with each other about problems in any meaningful way.

As previously described, patient and therapist form a self-selfobject unit in which selfobject needs are expressed and met on both sides, albeit to different degrees and in different ways. The therapist looks to the patient's responses for affirmation, consolidation and maintenance of the therapist's professional self. Needing to feel like the most important person in the room by being the channel through whom all family members communicate, or attempting to elicit explicit comments from patients about how helpful the treatment is, may reflect young and somewhat gross forms in which beginning therapists might express their need for affirmation, reminiscent of the way a young child might seek praise and attention. As the professional self grows firmer and the therapist gains in confidence and sophistication, the selfobject affirmation sought from the patient might be derived from the quiet pride and pleasure the therapist experiences in seeing his or her patient grow in inner strength, give voice to previously unexpressed ambitions, talents and ideals or take other steps forward, much as a parent takes pleasure in a growing child's increased capacity to move away and take on those things for him or herself which previously required the parent's active ministrations. These changes support the concept of a developmental progression in the selfobject experiences required for the sustenance of the professional self, with the form of these experiences maturing over the course of training.

The above case is also an example of reframing what otherwise might be more pejoratively viewed as countertransference. While the therapist's needs might indeed be intruding in a way that interferes with useful therapeutic technique in this situation, there is no need for the supervisor to respond negatively to this if the therapist's legitimate need for affirmation can be validated and channeled in a more appropriate direction. Understanding and accepting the therapist's experience of the situation mitigates defensiveness and helps the therapist change her behavior in a constructive way. Even more importantly, it provides the therapist with a vivid experience of the empathic mode of observation I am advocating she use with her patients.

These last vignettes, along with the examples presented earlier in this chapter, illustrate both the need of therapists in training for help managing their own experience and the way supervisors can effectively respond to this need. The goal is to help the therapist discuss feelings rather than act them out. The therapist's behavior is not seen as something bad, but rather as a solution to a problem. Using the empathic mode of inquiry, the supervisor helps the therapist identify what this problem is, along with the attempted solution, and then helps the person explore more adaptive alternatives. By proceeding in this fashion, the supervisor is able to provide a selfobject milieu sufficiently responsive to the therapist's emotional and cognitive needs for the central task of supervision to be achieved: the initiation of a structure-building process which will culminate in the therapist's acquisition of a cohesive professional self.

Notes

1 Others writing about supervision from a self psychological perspective make a similar point. Fuqua (1994) stated that the therapist must be the center of the supervisory process and the internal changes in his or her self structure are the focus. The way the supervisee experiences the patient is the supervisor's only viable starting point. P. Ornstein (1990) also emphasized the need to begin with an empathic immersion in the therapist's experience if one is to adequately evaluate interventions.

2 I have found it, incidentally, to be a fairly common occurrence that a therapist's reactions to supervisory input lead the therapist to become aware of other (countertransferential) feelings which had previously been out of his or her awareness.

References

Adler, G. (1984). Issues in the treatment of the borderline patient. In A. Goldberg & P. Stepansky (Eds.), *Kohut's legacy* (pp. 117–134). Hillsdale, NJ: Analytic Press.

Bacal, H. (1985). Optimal responsiveness and the therapeutic process. In A. Goldberg (Ed.), *Progress in self psychology* (Vol. 1, pp. 202–227). New York, NY: Guilford.

Bacal, H. (1990). The elements of a corrective selfobject experience. *Psychoanalytic Inquiry, 10*, 347–372.

Bacal, H. (1992, October). *The selfobject relationship in psychoanalytic treatment.* Paper presented at the 15th Annual Conference on the Psychology of the Self, Los Angeles, CA.

Barth, F.D. (1988). The patient as a selfobject: A form of countertransference. *Bulletin of the Menninger Clinic, 52*, 294–303.

Basch, M.F. (1988). *Understanding psychotherapy: The science behind the art.* New York, NY: Basic Books.

Brightman, B. (1984). Narcissistic issues in the training experience of the psychotherapist. *International Journal of Psychoanalytic Psychotherapy, 10*, 293–317.

Casement, P. (1985). *Learning from the patient.* New York, NY: Guilford Press.

Elson, M. (1989). The teacher as learner; the learner as teacher. In K. Field, B. Cohler, & G. Wool (Eds.), *Learning and education: Psychoanalytic perspectives* (pp. 789–808). Madison, CT: International Universities Press.

Friedman, D., & Kaslow, N. (1986). The development of professional identity in psychotherapists: Six stages in the supervision process. In F. Kaslow (Ed.), *Supervision and training: Models, dilemmas, and challenges* (pp. 29–49). New York, NY: Haworth Press.

Fuqua, P. (1994). Teaching, learning, and supervision. In A. Goldberg (Ed.), *A decade of progress: Progress in self psychology* (Vol. 10, pp. 79–98). Hillsdale, NJ: Analytic Press.

Gardner, J. (1991). The application of self psychology to brief psychotherapy. *Psychoanalytic Psychology, 8*, 477–500.

Gardner, J. (1995). Supervision of trainees: Tending the professional self. *Clinical Social Work Journal, 23*, 271–286.

Gediman, H., & Wolkenfeld, F. (1980). The parallelism phenomenon in psychoanalysis and supervision: Its reconsideration as a triadic system. *Psychoanalytic Quarterly, 49*, 234–255.

Kohut, H. (1959). Introspection, empathy and psychoanalysis. In P. Ornstein (Ed.), *The search for the self* (pp. 205–232). New York, NY: International Universities Press, 1978.

Kohut, H. (1977). *The restoration of the self.* New York, NY: International Universities Press.

Kohut, H. (1982). Introspection, empathy, and the semi-circle of mental health. *International Journal of Psychoanalysis, 63*, 395–407.

Kohut, H. (1984). *How does analysis cure?* Chicago, IL: University of Chicago Press.

Lichtenberg, J. (1988, October). *Rethinking the scope of the patient's transference and the therapist's countertransference.* Paper presented at the 11th Annual Conference on the Psychology of the Self, Washington, DC.

Miller, J. (1989, October). Can psychotherapy substitute for paychoanalysis? Paper presented to the 12th Annual Conference on the Psychology of the Self, San Francisco, CA.

Muslin, H., & Val, E. (1989). Supervision: A teaching-learning paradigm. In K. Field, B. Cohler, & G. Wool (Eds.), *Learning and education: Psychoanalytic perspectives* (pp. 159–179). Madison, CT: International Universities Press.

Ornstein, P. (1990). A self psychology view. *Psychoanalytic Inquiry*, *10*, 478–497.

Ornstein, P., & Ornstein, A. (1985). Clinical understanding and explaining: The empathic vantage point. In A. Goldberg (Ed.), *Progress in self psychology* (Vol. 1, pp. 43–61). New York, NY: Guilford Press.

Reams, R. (n.d.). *Selfobject transference in supervision*. Unpublished paper.

Sarnat, J. (1992). Supervision in relationship: Resolving the teach-treat controversy in psychoanalytic supervision. *Psychoanalytic Psychology*, *9*, 387–403.

Sloan, J. (1986). The empathic vantage point in supervision. In A. Goldberg (Ed.), *Progress in self psychology* (Vol. 2, pp. 188–211). New York, NY: Guilford Press.

Stolorow, R. (1983). Self psychology—A structural psychology. In J.D. Lichtenberg & S. Kaplan (Eds.), *Reflections on self psychology* (pp. 287–296). Hillsdale, NJ: Analytic Press.

Stolorow, R. (1986). Critical reflections on the theory of self psychology: An inside view. *Psychoanalytic Inquiry*, *6*, 387–402.

Terman, D. (1988). Optimum frustration: Structuralization and the therapeutic process. In A. Goldberg (Ed.), *Learning from Kohut: Progress in self psychology* (Vol. 4, pp. 113–126). Hillsdale, NJ: Analytic Press.

Terman, D. (1989). Therapeutic change: Perspectives of self psychology. *Psychoanalytic Inquiry*, *9*, 88–100.

Tolpin, P. (1988). Optimal affective engagement: The analyst's role in therapy. In A. Goldberg (Ed.), *Learning from Kohut: Progress in self psychology* (Vol. 4, pp. 160–167). Hillsdale, NJ: Analytic Press.

Winnicott, D.W. (1965). *The maturational processes and the facilitating environment*. New York, NY: International Universities Press.

Wolf, E.S. (1983). Empathy and countertransference. In A. Goldberg (Ed.), *The future of psychoanalysis* (pp. 309–326). New York, NY: International Universities Press.

Wolf, E.S. (1988). *Treating the self: Elements of clinical self psychology*. New York, NY: Guilford Press.

Part Two

Chapter 5

Interpretation and Development

Starting with this chapter, the following three chapters originated as responses to the writings of others, to explicate, expand on and dialogue with their ideas. In my discussion here of Richard Geist's paper on interpretation as a carrier of selfobject functions, I start by offering a description of how the concept of interpretation has evolved since both Freud and Kohut. I then clarify how the theory of development offered by Kohut and elaborated by Marian Tolpin dovetails with how Geist understands the mutative power of interpretation and how this perspective differs from earlier views offered by self psychologists. In keeping with my focus on translating theory to practice, in this piece I also elaborate the process by which we help people shift from a focus on external people and events to a focus on their internal experience. As will be elaborated even further in my discussion of self-agency in the next chapter, I see such shifts as the heart of what gives individuals the power to impact and make lasting changes in their lives. Experience-near examples are offered to help the reader understand abstract concepts such as connectedness.

This paper was published in 2020 as "Discussion of Richard Geist's 'Interpretation as Carrier of Selfobject Functions: Catalyzing Inborn Potential" in Psychoanalysis, Self and Context, *Volume 15.*

Since I find myself in essential agreement with what Geist (2020a) has written, I thought what might be most helpful in a discussion would be to contextualize and highlight some of his ideas. In terms of context, I'd like to comment briefly on how the concept of interpretation has evolved over time and also say a little bit more about development.

Interpretation is a foundational concept that every psychoanalytic writer and theory since Freud has addressed in one way or another. Kohut originally tried to correct what he saw as the over-emphasis on the explanatory

DOI: 10.4324/9781003491453-7

function of interpretation by adding a focus on the understanding dimension. For Kohut, interpretation involved both understanding *and* explaining (Kohut, 1977; P. Ornstein & Ornstein, 1985). Although he began to allude to the importance of the relational context in determining the effectiveness of interpretations, for Kohut the interpretation of selfobject transference remained the main vehicle of therapeutic action in his theory (Kohut, 1984).

In the years since Kohut, we have seen a dramatic expansion of our understanding of both the meaning of interpretation and the place of interpretation in our work. The dialogue regarding this topic has often been cast in terms of opposites: interpretation versus relationship; insight versus (new) experience; the cognitive versus the affective; or the verbal and explicit versus the nonverbal, procedural and implicit. Reams have been written about these distinctions. Yet we have now come to understand these as false dichotomies: that any verbal interpretation is laden with relational, affective and procedural meaning; that all interpretation occurs in an intersubjectively constituted relational context; and that often new understanding is perceived and communicated outside of conscious awareness altogether, without ever getting verbally articulated.

At the 29th Annual Conference on the Psychology of the Self, in 2006, a panel on interpretation included papers (later published) by Anna Ornstein (2009) and Shelley Doctors (2009). Like Geist, both of them saw interpretation as an ongoing, dialogic process, and both were concerned with how enduring change is facilitated in the clinical situation, i.e., how new ways of being and relating become enduring aspects of the patient's self—whether self is conceptualized in terms of internal psychic structure, functional capacities or organizations of experience.

There are many overlapping points between what they wrote and what Geist is saying. They turned to therapeutic action and described interpretations as communicating understanding (Ornstein) or illuminating meaning (Doctors). They talked about the human presence of the therapist and the intersubjective context, mutual influence and bidirectional nature of the relationship, as Geist does too. But Geist is adding something different and new here. What neither Doctors or Ornstein nor anyone else has talked or written about in quite the same way is the role of interpretations in catalyzing a potential that is *already there* internally.

We've all known and been saying for quite a while that interpretations serve selfobject functions. So at first glance, reading Geist's paper, we might wonder, "Didn't we already know all this? that good interpretations have selfobject functions? that understanding evokes a selfobject experience of validation or mirroring? and explaining evokes an idealizing selfobject experience of organizing and making sense out of our subjective reality?" What is he adding here? At its most basic, what he is adding is a different way of conceptualizing the therapeutic action of interpretation. By describing interpretations as catalyzing something already internal, rather than interpretations facilitating a process of taking in something from the outside, Geist is redefining the essence of their mutative power. He also elaborates what he thinks facilitates being able to make effective interpretations, and I'll come back to that in a moment. But first, a few words about development.

Geist opens his article with a quote from Marian Tolpin (1986), which he then sets out to elaborate, about how interpretations are carriers of selfobject functions that foster further internalization. I think it would be helpful here to bring in a little bit more about Tolpin's developmental theory, which dovetails particularly well with what Geist goes on to say. She may not have gotten around to elaborating the original idea Geist has picked up, but she did elaborate a particular view of development that creates, in my opinion, a very natural bridge to what he wrote.

Tolpin (1987) described development as an interdependence of givens and experience; the idea that the child's own resources and the parents' selfobject functions act as magnets for development (her metaphor). In her 1986 paper on a different baby, she put it this way: "A primary psychological tendency (a given) propels the normal baby to establish selfobject ties. By offering adequate selfobject responses to the baby's connecting initiatives, parents and others insure that this tendency will continue through the successive stages of development" (p. 124).

I think this is exactly what Geist is describing in terms of therapeutic action. It's the idea of that same inborn potential and that similarly catalyzing effect of the therapist's selfobject-rich interpretations that come together to create forward movement and change. Basically, he's defining for us what he thinks makes interpretations so important (as he says, in all treatments) and what makes them mutative.

Geist also brings up disruption and repair. He says these cycles are useful for transmuting internalization, but not required for internalizations to occur. This reminds me of our move from optimal frustration to optimal response, the recognition that self-cohesion can be strengthened, or structure building occur, without frustration (Bacal, 1985; Terman, 1988).

When Wolf (1988) talked about disruption/repair, he focused on disruptions in the transference. The way he explained it was that experience is organized in particular ways; disruptions lead to a disorganization. The individual will then reorganize in the context of what is at hand. If what is at hand is a therapist who empathically understands and validates the person's experience as legitimate rather than a parent who blames, withdraws or retaliates, the person will reorganize in a way that promotes a more robust sense of self, with increased capacities for self-righting and the ability to embrace their own subjective experience as legitimate and valid.

In Geist's example of Carrie, who felt shamed when her boyfriend abandoned her right after having sex, something similar happened—there was a disruption and repair—but not primarily in the transference. By helping Carrie understand how her experience with her boyfriend had resonated with and evoked a long history of such shaming encounters with her mother, she went from a state of disorganization to feeling more organized and able to manage her affect. In other words, with Geist's help she reorganized in a new way—not by taking in or internalizing her therapist's more validating, less shaming stance than figures in her past had taken, but by his mobilizing her own internal capacity and potential for self-righting.

I think it's important to note that the interpretations that Geist describes as mutative and catalyzing inborn potentials work powerfully when (and perhaps because) they strike the patient as profoundly correct, leading to the strong sense of physical and emotional relief his patients reported. Kohut (1984) was undoubtedly referencing this kind of depth in his famous comment about times when his "rightness" was superficial, while his patients' rightness was profound. I do not mean we need to know such correctness at the outset, rather than having it emerge through dialogue. Over and over Geist offers his interpretations with a question mark—could it be, is it possible—and an invitation to correct what he's said if it feels off. But when he hits the mark, the patient feels deeply and accurately understood and is thereby able to make a new kind of organizing sense out of their otherwise distressed feelings.

This is where the concepts of connectedness and permeable boundaries come in (Geist, 2008, 2009). They facilitate deep empathic immersion in the patient's experience via the therapist's deep empathic immersion and resonance with his or her own internal experience. As one person said to me on a particular occasion, "When you spoke I felt like your breath came through me, like you not only knew how I felt, but felt how I felt." This is the essence of connectedness and permeable boundaries, without which we don't evoke the kind of deep selfobject experience that catalyzes internal growth in the way Geist is describing.

Speaking of connectedness and permeable boundaries, sometimes people have trouble grasping exactly what these terms mean. Geist tries to illustrate these concepts in all his clinical writings and vignettes. But let me add one very concrete, visual image by way of analogy. Picture the 10- or 12-month-old child, taking his or her first, wobbly steps toward an adult several yards away. That child is supported by the arms reaching out for her until she makes it across the divide into the loving, proud embrace of the adult. Those arms become part of the child's own body— *her* balance, mobility and capacity to remain upright—while crossing the room. If the parent's arms drop midway, the child is likely to fall. This is simply an analogy in physical terms of what Geist is describing in emotional terms.

Let me come back now to how these ideas are relevant to creating the mutative power of interpretations Geist is describing. What comes across in the vignettes in this paper, and in all of Geist's papers, is the way he is "in it" with his patients. With his more difficult patient, Judy, for example, he lets himself *be* her (internally) in order to grasp her experience of him. With all his patients, by consistently sharing his subjectivity and allowing himself to be vulnerable, he promotes the kind of connectedness that enables his understanding. Conveying that understanding via interpretation then catalyzes a process of self understanding in his patients. And it is that *self understanding* that is organizing and structure building. By structure building, I mean enduring. When we reorganize our experience of events in the present and past, it carries forward to new understandings and organizations of experiences in the future.

Intersubjectivists refer to such changes as the transformation of previously unconscious organizing principles (e.g., Stolorow, Brandchaft, & Atwood, 1987). Once we reorganize our experience of the present and past in new ways, we are able to perceive and experience ourselves and others in the future in similarly new ways. The same goes for increased capacities for self-righting and affect management as enduring, internal capacities.

The last thing I want to underscore is Geist's point about focusing on intrapsychic space between patient and therapist rather than the interpersonal. He may name his behavior in the session, but always as a preface to a statement about some way what he said or did was experienced internally by the patient, and what that in turn then triggered. Many of our patients come to us with a focus on how the actions of others and external forces are the source of their troubles, whether it's a bad boss, a bully husband, a demanding parent, a callous boyfriend or girlfriend or, in the treatment, an unavailable or misattuned therapist. And the corollary is little awareness of how these people and actions evoke and resonate with old hurts and memories that amplify the current experience. Noxious or distressing external events trigger internal reactions, and it is the combination of the two, what the other does (or fails to do) and what we're doing with it, that ultimately determines our experience. The potential for change resides in recognizing and claiming ownership over the part that is internal.

As Geist emphasized in quoting Paul Ornstein, our job in general and how we understand growth and change has to do with helping people shift from what is external to understanding what, initially out of their awareness, is going on internally. Geist's examples illustrate how this process unfolds, which is in turn, I think, the point of his article. It starts first by connectedness, the establishment of a "we" or us, and then by offering interpretations with selfobject functions that can be used and metabolized by the patient to mobilize their inherent potentials for greater self-organization and regulation. Being able to see that it is their own internal reactions that most powerfully determine their subjective experience of events gives patients enormous new power to impact and, ultimately, change their lives.

Most articles in our journals and presentations at our conferences are, in the end, concerned with therapeutic action, the question of what makes treatment work, what enables us to help people make enduring changes. We can thank Dick Geist for offering us a new perspective on this most important question, by sharing his thoughts on how interpretation as a carrier of selfobject functions catalyzes inborn potential.

That said, I'd like to end by posing a (perhaps radical) question for Geist and us all: Why does it matter to think of it this way? I've tried to highlight what Geist is saying that is different and new, but what do we gain by this different way of understanding the therapeutic action of interpretation? What do we lose by *not* thinking about it this way? How does it impact what we do, and what is the yield clinically? Once again, I thank Dick Geist for offering us, as ever, such a clinically rich and interesting set of ideas to consider.[1]

Note

1 For Geist's response to these questions, see Geist (2020b).

References

Bacal, H. (1985). Optimal responsiveness and the therapeutic process. In A. Goldberg (Ed.), *Progress in self psychology* (pp. 202–227). New York, NY: Guilford Press.

Doctors, S. (2009). Interpretation as a relational process. *International Journal of Psychoanalytic Self Psychology, 4*, 449–465.

Gardner, J. (2020). Discussion of George Hagman's "Self-agency: Context and freedom in psychoanalysis." *Psychoanalysis, Self, and Context, 15*, 40–46.

Gardner, J. (2020). Discussion of Richard Geist's "Interpretation as carrier of selfobject functions: Catalyzing inborn potential." *Psychoanalysis, Self, and Context, 15*, 40–46.

Geist, R. (2008). Connectedness, permeable boundaries, and the development of the self: Therapeutic implications. *International Journal of Psychoanalytic Self Psychology, 3*, 129–152.

Geist, R. (2009). Empathy, connectedness, and the evolution of boundaries in self psychological treatment. *International Journal of Psychoanalytic Self Psychology, 4*, 165–180.

Geist, R. (2020a). Interpretation as carrier of selfobject functions: Catalyzing inborn potential. *Psychonanalysis, Self, and Context, 15*, 338–347.

Geist, R. (2020b). Response to Jill Gardner's discussion of interpretation as a carrier of selfobject functions. *Psychoanalysis, Self and Context, 15*, 353–355.

Kohut, H. (1977). *The restoration of the self.* New York, NY: International Universities Press.

Kohut, H. (1984). *How does analysis cure?* Chicago, IL: University of Chicago Press.

Ornstein, A. (2009). Do words still matter? Further comments on the interpretive process and the theory of change. *International Journal of Psychoanalytic Self Psychology, 4*, 466–484.

Ornstein, P., & Ornstein, A. (1985). Clinical understanding and explaining: The empathic vantage point. In A. Goldberg (Ed.), *Progress in self psychology* (pp. 43–61). New York, NY: Guilford Press.

Stolorow, R., Brandchaft, B., & Atwood, G. (1987). *Psychoanalytic treatment: An intersubjective approach.* New York, NY: Routledge.

Terman, D. (1988). Optimum frustration: Structuralization and the therapeutic process. In A. Goldberg (Ed.), *Progress in self psychology* (4th ed., pp. 113–125). Hillsdale, NJ: Analytic Press.

Tolpin, M. (1986). The self and its selfobjects: A different baby. In A. Goldberg (Ed.), *Progress in self psychology* (2nd ed., pp. 115–128). New York, NY: Guilford Press.

Tolpin, M. (1987). Discussion of Margaret Black's The analyst's stance: Transferential implications of technical orientation. *The Annual of Psychoanalysis, 15*, 159–164. Madison, CT: International Universities Press.

Wolf, E. (1988). *Treating the self.* New York, NY: Guilford Press.

Chapter 6

Self-agency, Defense and the Forward Edge

In this discussion of George Hagman's paper on self-agency, I expand and elaborate upon our understanding of defense, the paradoxical ways early coping strategies can both impede and express a sense of agency and the role of forward edge interpretation in restoring both ownership of one's choices and a sense of personal agency. In discussing Hagman's case, I illustrate some of the principles I outlined in the previous chapters on brief treatment by drawing from his clinical examples, again seeking to link theory and practice. Similarly, I clarify how it is the combination of noxious external events and the internal reactions they trigger that ultimately determines our experience and becomes an important focus of treatment. Finally, I discuss how a sense of agency can be both threatened and restored in the broader context of historical and political events.

This paper was published in 2020 as "Discussion of George Hagman's 'Self-Agency: Context and Freedom in Psychoanalysis'" in Psychoanalysis, Self and Context, *Volume 15.*

Hagman's (2020) article on self-agency struck me initially for two reasons. First, it felt very clinically relevant and true, resonating as it did with my experience of what many of my patients looked like, sounded like and struggled with. Second, it created an umbrella, in a sense, for so many other clinical concepts that have been central to the evolution of our theory and among the most useful to me personally. The following discussion clarifies and expands upon Hagman's ideas, while elaborating some additional ones of my own regarding defense and agency.

Hagman places a sense of personal agency at the heart of self-development and self-experience. He elaborates Kohut's concept of the self as a center of initiative by emphasizing that we also need to be a center of creative action. Helping children, and later our patients, develop a sense of

DOI: 10.4324/9781003491453-8

confidence in their own agency, he tells us, involves more than affective attunement. Rather, it requires empathy to the self as a dynamic, evolving actor, recognizing and affirming the child's (or later patient's) creative thought, feeling and resourcefulness.

Agency requires acting on the basis of internal experience, one's own thoughts, feelings, needs, intentions and preferred choices. But in order to do this, we need to know what our internal experience is. Developmentally, this requires recognition, validation and encouragement of what comes from the inside out; that is, what emanates internally. Children require the help of adults to name and organize their feelings and intentions. We say things like, "Oh, that loud noise *scared* you!" or "You're piling the blocks so high. You're making something very tall, maybe like a tower?"

Children are also strongly motivated to have control of the world around them, both human and non-human. Wolf (1988) described this as a need for efficacy selfobject experience, the ability to make a dent on the world. He quotes Lichtenberg's (1983) observation that infants will maintain their interest in watching a series of blinking lights longer when they can control the pattern of the lights than when that pattern is completely random. In a related vein, Basch (1988) saw a sense of competence as a primary motivation in human behavior and the basis of self-esteem. This intuitively rings true. When we experience ourselves as competent and effective actors, whatever the situation, we generally feel good about ourselves. When we feel incompetent at something or unable to manage effectively, our self-esteem goes down.

In addition to describing the normal and optimal developmental conditions for agency to mature and solidify, Hagman describes how this process can be derailed, disrupted or usurped under conditions of early trauma. Once they have experienced such trauma, children will go to great lengths to protect themselves from impingement, empathic failure or retraumatization. But the prolonged state of dependence and helplessness of the human child also makes our early bond with caregivers essential for survival. So, when the environment, in any number of ways, does not lend itself to recognition, validation and acceptance of what is authentically the child's internal experience (volitions, perceptions, etc.), the child will take whatever emergency measures he or she can find to protect *both* the nascent sense of self *and* the bond with the needed caregiver. This is the breeding ground or origin of what has traditionally been called defense and resistance.

From a self psychological perspective, we see these measures as adaptations to vulnerability and ways to protect the self from the retraumatization of empathic failure. Changing the moral tone with which such maneuvers were historically approached in analytic theory, Wolf (1988) suggested we think of them not as defense or resistance but instead as "obligatory measures of self protection." A classic example is Brandchaft's (2007) concept of pathological accommodation, which is generally a surrender of self, authenticity, agency and initiative in order to protect the bond with the parent. If the parent cannot adjust to and accept the child's subjective reality, the child will adopt the parent's reality to preserve the needed tie.

Hagman's case of David illustrates beautifully how these adaptations become manifest in the transference, not, as he notes, as resistance but as continued attempts to protect the self through methods that have become firmly established for doing so. David seeks protection against coercive intrusion, a feared and dreaded repeat of his childhood experience of impingement or usurpation of his agency and authentic experience by his mother. Shutting Hagman out by "doing his own analysis" echoes his early attempts to maintain control by retreating from the dinner table to his bedroom.

It is important to realize that these adaptations are active, creative efforts to preserve both self and needed ties and are, paradoxically, therefore expressions of exactly what is being threatened—the sense of agency. In order to help someone like this, it is crucial that we see this healthy, forward edge in the patient's motivation and behavior, what Marian Tolpin (2002) described as the tendril of health entwined in what otherwise might be seen as simply pathology.

Again, Hagman illustrates this when he tells David that his sense of control in the treatment is understandably important, that the only way to be safely in control at home was to go off by himself, manage his feelings and figure out what to do. So, for David, to let Hagman and his words in is to open himself up once again to having his subjective experience crushed under the weight of the other person's perspective.

Michael Basch (1995) stressed the importance of focusing on a patient's strengths. When Hagman tells David that his effort to cope "allowed him to be in charge and to organize and manage his inner and outer worlds in a way which served his need for control and protection," he is doing exactly that. One of the hallmarks of our self psychological approach to interpretation is to place our emphasis on what our patients are striving to do rather than what they are trying to avoid and what is right, i.e., healthy, about their choices, rather than what is wrong or pathological. Hagman's forward edge interpretation here enables David to feel understood in depth, offers belated recognition and affirmation of his creative act of self-preservation and facilitates his dawning awareness of his own role in authoring the actions that now cause him great difficulty. This last point is a central aspect of therapeutic action that Hagman emphasizes in his article.

The protective maneuvers and adaptations, as life-saving as they may have been originally, have an underside of great cost. Again paradoxically, the very expressions of agency that created protection against threats to agency in the patient's past become huge impediments to agency in the adult patient's present. A hallmark of agency is the ability to adapt flexibly to new contexts in an active and proactive way. However, the templates we develop about self-with-other operate largely out of our conscious awareness. We develop assumptions about how things work in the interpersonal world that on the one hand provide structure, while on other limit our perceptions, expectations, actions and choice—i.e., our agency.

Many different names have been given to these assumptions or structures: working models (Bowlby, 1969), RIGS (Stern, 1985), emotional convictions (Orange, 1995), invariant organizing principles (Stolorow, Brandchaft, & Atwood, 1987). Unless reexamined, usually under the microscope of psychotherapy, these implicit assumptions become rigid and unchanging, as do the adaptations for dealing with trauma, like David's. Ultimately this creates a loss of flexibility and creativity, both of which are essential for maintaining a sense of agency. Much of the work of therapy involves liberating the patient's capacity for self-agency from the shackles of previous adaptations that are no longer relevant, required or useful.

Because our patients generally start out with no awareness of these dynamics and phenomena, the things that on a deep level propel their behavior and inform and constrict their experience, it is imperative to stay initially with what is consciously available and not prematurely threaten what has been their best or only way of protecting themselves. This is just what Hagman does with David when he restrains his own desire to interpret and allows David to keep him shut out, respecting David's self-agency in order to cultivate an environment of trust, free of the threat of coercion or impingement. The goal, as Hagman describes, is to enable David eventually to see that his difficulties are not a product of external forces, but rather of internal choices made long ago that have become rigid and constraining, impeding the very goals of self-determination and agency they once served to protect.

Joye Weisel-Barth (2009), writing about agency in the context of determinism, described how patients often present themselves as being at the mercy of powerful forces, unable to make choices and living their lives passively. "Like stones in a rushing stream, such people feel the current of life as something out there, eddying around or washing over them, rather than as a process in which they actively participate, a process that reflects creative choice, action, and responsibility" (p. 294). Hagman similarly describes people who have undergone a derailment of agency in childhood as experiencing their suffering as out of their control and their own feelings, thoughts and desires as invalid or worthless.

The passivity and helplessness that both Weisel-Barth and Hagman describe feel very accurate in terms of my experience of how our patients often present and describe their own experience. They ride in the passenger seat of their lives, metaphorically, only able to go where driven by others rather than getting behind the wheel and charting their own course. They can describe what troubles them—their pain or their inability to realize certain goals—but they often have no sense of either how they contribute to creating and sustaining the problems that thwart and trouble them or how they could possibly make it different. For some people, the idea of attending to internal experience at all—thoughts, feelings, needs, desires, perceptions—is entirely novel. External forces, such as the bad boss, the bully husband, the demanding parent or the defiant child, are presented initially as the source of problems, rather than the source being in the patient's reactions and response to these people, the felt or automatic imperative to accommodate, or withdraw, or defy, and so forth.

It is not that circumstances or other people in the patient's life are not difficult. They often are. One way I've sometimes tried to help people understand their own role in reacting to a difficult person's behavior is to say, "Yes, their behavior was certainly and understandably upsetting. But it was also just the spark or match; inside you is a fuel tank which that match then ignited into something explosive and overwhelming."[1] The point of the metaphor is that noxious external events trigger internal reactions, and it is the *combination* of the two (what the other does and what we're doing with it) that ultimately determines our experience. Subjective experience is always both contextually and intersubjectively constituted. The potential for agency (and change) resides in recognizing and claiming ownership over the part that is internal. In Hagman's clinical example, David expresses this beautifully when he says, "I want to get to the point where I can stay at the table. That their abuse and laughter doesn't matter. That's their problem. So I can just stay and enjoy my meal. That's what I want." In other words, he sees that the needed change is in what *he* does, in changing his response internally and then behaviorally, rather than in trying to change the thing that triggered it.

This is exactly what I see so many people struggling with. They can't figure out how to get out from under the circumstances or people that they perceive as constraining them, to get to the point where, like David, they can be separate enough that what the other person does doesn't matter, that they can express their own sense of agency regardless.[2] In order to do so, they need to recognize and claim their own participation in constructing their experience; they need to understand the positive role such behavior played for them historically; and they need to reexamine whether yesterday's solutions are still necessary or helpful today. Adults potentially have options and resources that children don't. New solutions may need to be forged and old ones abandoned, in order to live a more meaningful and fulfilling life.

One author I read noted that someone can intentionally send you poison, but if you do not swallow it, it will not hurt you. David wants to be separate enough not to swallow the poison of his mother's criticism, but rather to ignore her and enjoy his meal instead. The recognition of this possibility, along with the experience of having found a sense of safety in his relationship with Hagman, is what opens a pathway to resolving his presenting problem. David feared he would be chronically alone because his inability to trust any woman would lead him always to withdraw and reject her.[3] Together, David and Hagman found their way to a new, potentially different solution and, therefore, a potentially different outcome.

In Hagman's paper and in this discussion, we have focused on the developmental derailment of a sense of agency and its restoration. The clinical case illustrates how such a person might behave in the transference and what would be needed to resolve the presenting problems. Before ending this discussion, I would like to pick up on one other aspect of the topic we have not discussed. Sander (2004) noted that maintaining a sense of agency is an ongoing, life-long process. New contexts, including historical and political events, can challenge our sense of agency.

In the United States, clinicians saw this after the election of Donald Trump in 2016. Many patients described a profound sense of helplessness and despair. One physician I see felt his sense of agency and control so threatened that he began thinking about where he could possibly emigrate to practice medicine, fearing that life in the US might become so intolerable that he and his family might have to leave the country entirely. Others complained of a loss of control over things that they held very dear, particularly certain core values. As the Trump presidency progressed, his base consolidated and all branches of government became increasingly controlled by people of a similar political persuasion, the challenge to a sense of agency among those who felt differently only intensified. Some were mobilized to greater action; others fell deeper into a sense of doom and impotence. The United States is not alone in facing upheaval of the established order. Much of the world is struggling with great and far-reaching changes. Neither we nor our patients are separate from these broader contexts of experience. Well-being, in these circumstances, is highly dependent on finding ways to maintain our sense of agency, even in the face of circumstances we may have limited power to control. Whatever the ultimate outcomes, our sense of self in these larger contexts is colored greatly by whether or not we retain a sense of personal agency, the sense that we can make choices and take actions that try to make a difference, in our own lives and/or in the lives of others.

The work of Victor Frankl is instructive here. A psychiatrist who survived Nazi death camps, Frankl (1959) noted that the people who made the best adjustments after that traumatic experience were those who maintained some sense of agency during their imprisonment. Frankl described a "circle of concern," which included everything one might worry about, and within that circle a smaller "circle of influence," which included everything one might be able to do something about. In a concentration camp, the circle of concern was enormous: Will I survive? will I ever seen my family again? are they all right? will I get enough to eat? will I freeze? will I die of illness even before they kill me? and on and on. In contrast, the circle of influence and control was miniscule. Yet even in that extreme environment, where almost nothing seemed within a prisoner's power to impact, there was a place for acts of personal choice and agency. Given a meager portion of food in the morning, would one eat it all at once, in order to have enough energy and strength to make it through the day? or save it for evening, in order to have a reward and something to look forward to after working all day? or eat half at the beginning and half at the end of the day? It doesn't sound like much of a choice, but it is a choice nevertheless, a scrap of personal agency that in the end made a difference among those who survived, a difference in their ability to move forward in life after such terrible trauma.[4]

Fortunately, most of our patients are not currently in such desperate straits. But many were and are in very challenging, abusive or daunting situations. And I think their challenge and our challenge is the same: Helping them to develop, restore and/or maintain the sense of agency that I believe, in agreement with Hagman, is crucial to robust self-experience and the sense of well-being.

Notes

1 Such fuel tanks are, of course, created by the old hurts and memories that are evoked by, resonate with and amplify the current experience.
2 To be clear, agency and separateness, as described here, are not the same as autonomy. Any absolute autonomy, in an intersubjectively constituted world, is neither possible nor the goal of development.
3 This, incidentally, is the real meaning of Anna Ornstein's concept of the dread to repeat (1974). While often taken as meaning the dread to repeat traumatic experiences, the fear she described was actually of repeating the old defensive solutions and adaptations that no longer were suited to current realities and goals.
4 Anna Ornstein (1985) also has noted, in this context, that manifest behavioral passivity in this environment should not necessarily be taken as a lack of agency, nor as evidence of helplessness or capitulation. "Survival required a great deal of activity and resistance in all aspects of camp life: not to fall asleep when standing in line for hours, not to sit down when totally exhausted, not to eat the piece of bread that was to last for a whole day. All required extraordinary levels of activity" (p. 113).

References

Basch, M.F. (1988). *Understanding psychotherapy: The science behind the art*. New York, NY: Basic Books.

Basch, M.F. (1995). *Doing brief psychotherapy*. New York, NY: Basic Books.

Bowlby, J. (1969). *Attachment and loss, volume 1*. New York, NY: Basic Books.

Brandchaft, B. (2007). Systems of pathological accommodation and change in analysis. *Psychoanalytic Psychology, 24*, 667–687.

Frankl, V. (1959). *Man's search for meaning*. Boston, MA: Beacon Press.

Gardner, J. (2020). Discussion of George Hagman's "Self-agency: Context and freedom in psychoanalysis." *Psychoanalysis, Self, and Context, 15*, 348–352.

Hagman, G. (2020). Self-agency: Context and freedom in psychoanalysis, *Psychoanalysis, Self and Context, 15*, 33–39.

Lichtenberg, J. (1983). *Psychoanalysis and infant research*. Hillsdale, NJ: Analytic Press.

Orange, D. (1995). *Emotional understanding: Studies in psychoanalytic epistemology*. New York, NY: Guilford Press.

Ornstein, A. (1974). The dread to repeat and the new beginning: A contribution to the psychoanalysis of the narcissistic personality disorders. *Annual of Psychoanalysis*, *2*, 231–248.

Ornstein, A. (1985). Survival and recovery. *Psychoanalytic Inquiry*, *5*, 99–130.

Sander, L. (2004). *Living systems, evolving consciousness, and the emerging person: A selection of papers from the life and work of Louis Sander* (G. Amadei & I. Bianchi, Eds.). New York, NY: The Analytic Press.

Stern, D. (1985). *The interpersonal world of the infant: A view from psychoanalysis and developmental psychology*. New York, NY: Basic Books.

Stolorow, R., Brandchaft, B., & Atwood, G. (1987). *Psychoanalytic treatment: An intersubjective approach*. New York, NY: The Analytic Press.

Tolpin, M. (2002). Doing psychoanalysis of normal development: Forward edge transferences. *Progress in Self Psychology*, *18*, 167–190.

Weisel-Barth, J. (2009). Stuck: Choice and agency in psychoanalysis. *International Journal of Psychoanalytic Self Psychology*, *4*, 288–312.

Wolf, E.S. (1988). *Treating the self*. New York, NY: Guilford Press.

Chapter 7

Transference and the Self

Where my discussion of Geist's paper gave me an opportunity to elaborate ideas about interpretation and development, and my discussion of Hagman's paper gave me an opportunity to elaborate my ideas about defense, agency and the forward edge, in my discussion of the paper by Barry Magid, James Fosshage and Estelle Shane on Relational Self Psychology, I elaborate ideas about transference. In contrast to the chapters in Part One of this book, the discussion here is written with a full appreciation of the latest and most contemporary developments in self psychology and intersubjectivity theory. However, I raise a concern that the authors do not more sufficiently elaborate the through lines of our theory that remain core and guiding principles. I elaborate thoughts about transference because I see our understanding of this topic as central to the issue of asymmetry in the therapeutic relationship. Also, in the context of our contemporary emphasis on mutual influence and co-creation in the analytic relationship, a focus on transference guides us to the steadfast focus on internal experience which has been at the heart of all the previous chapters.

This paper was published in 2021 as "Whither the Self in Relational Self Psychology? A Comment on Magid, Fosshage & Shane's Article" in Psychoanalysis, Self and Context, *Volume 16.*

In their historical review which culminates in what Magid, Fosshage, and Shane (2021) have called Relational Self Psychology, the authors trace innovations since Kohut's death in two areas: the concept of self and the concept of how change is created in psychoanalytic treatment. In this brief comment, I'd like to raise some questions about the first of these topics, the concept of self.

DOI: 10.4324/9781003491453-9

While it is true that Kohut wrote about the "nuclear self" as a kind of structural entity, poised to unfold in the context of adequate selfobject responsiveness, the very notion of a selfobject matrix made Kohut's self always a relational concept. A two-person assumption is inherent in the concepts of both selfobject experience and selfobject transference. Over time, others continued Kohut's project by making explicit what he had suggested only implicitly.

In a memorable exchange during the 2006 International Conference on the Psychology of the Self, Marian Tolpin, responding to a plenary presentation by Dick Geist, complained that people were talking about Kohut having a one-person theory, when in fact his notion of self was always a two-person concept. Geist famously replied that while those who worked directly with him or his small group of close supporters were aware that clinically Kohut worked from a two-person perspective, those of us who did not work directly with him could only go by his theoretical writing, which was in one-person terms.

In regard to Magid et al., I have a similar concern in relation to how these senior clinicians actually think and practice *vs* what they have written in this article. My concern is not with what the authors said, but with what they did not elaborate more explicitly. They carefully document the evolution and changes in both our concepts of self and our concept of how change comes about through the psychoanalytic relationship and process. In this endeavor, they very helpfully bring together many disparate ideas and clarify the connections between them. They do not with similar detail describe the continuities, however. In their focus on what's new and what's changed, do we ignore something that is old and still true, even necessary? After citing a number of postmodern psychoanalytic theorists, they state:

> How far beyond Kohut's original contributions these formulations take us is an open question, one which asks us to balance our shifting experience of innovation with an acknowledgement of the continuity embodied by the series of steps that brought us to where we are today. 'Relational self psychology' is our attempt to encompass the significant changes in perspective that have emerged since Kohut's death with a full appreciation of his core insights that continue to guide us into the future.

(p. 4)

I do not find in the article any further description of what the authors believe those continuing core insights are. In this vein, what I particularly would like to hear more about is what the authors believe remains true and relevant in our earlier conceptions of self, as it impacts their own clinical work, especially *vis-à-vis* the role of selfobject experience and selfobject transference. At this point in the evolution of our theory, most of us would agree that the sense of self is intersubjectively constituted in specific relational contexts. But when we encounter a patient, that person enters with something that is more than that which is co-constructed with us. This is the part that remains unelaborated in their article, as they focus on systems and bi-directional influences.

Based on previous experience, the patient's self and experience have become patterned and organized, *vis-à-vis* both affect and relationships. Whether we refer to that patterning as working models (Bowlby, 1988), patterns of expectation (Beebe & Lachmann, 1988), organizing principles (e.g., Stolorow, Atwood, & Brandchaft, 1987), emotional convictions (Orange, 1996), implicit relational knowing (Bruschweiler-Stern et al., 2002; Lyons-Ruth, 1999) or attractor states (Thelen & Smith, 1994), something is there already when the patient first walks through the door. Based on this previous patterning, there are multiple dimensions of transference that may be evoked in the treatment relationship: forward or trailing edge (Kohut, 1984; Tolpin, 2002); needed or repeated (Stern, 1994, 2017); selfobject or repetitive/conflictual (Stolorow et al., 1987); old-old or new-new (Shane, Shane, & Gales, 1997) and so forth. Who the therapist is and what the therapist does will evoke some of these and not others. But it is, nevertheless, all potentially there in the patient to be evoked or catalyzed.

A new patient enters our encounter with hopes, needs and wishes, previously met and unmet: for acceptance, support, validation, guidance, inclusion. He or she brings fears, dreads and negative expectations: of misattunement, abandonment, intrusion, retaliation, criticism. The patient also comes with defenses and adaptations: accommodation, withdrawal, aggression. And with symptoms in the service of self regulation, whether for calming or enlivening: eating disorders, chemical and behavioral addictions, obsessions and compulsions and so forth. As suggested above, any of these aspects of the person may become manifest in the transference. Although Magid et al. mention the variety of ways transference has been conceptualized by different theorists, I think they emphasize the fluidity of self organization at the expense of the continuity of it. To paraphrase Judy

Teicholz, as she once felicitously put it in a journal club post, are we at risk of losing the subject in intersubjectivity?

In their summary statement about the nature of self, Magid et al. say we are moving

> toward a recognition that we use the word *self* to encompass a variety of conceptual and subjective phenomena, encompassing both our subjective, conscious experience of identity and agency, as well as describing metapsychological levels of cohesion or fragmentation, capacities for affect regulation and attunement, and relational patterns of attachment and expectation.
>
> (p. 18)

Certainly, affect regulation and relational patterns remain central to our understanding of self. Socarides and Stolorow (1984–1985) described selfobject functions as pertaining fundamentally to the integration of affect; Michael Basch (1988) described affect management as the heart of psychotherapy; and multiple authors have cited the expansion of relational patterns and possibilities as the way self experience is transformed in successful treatment (e.g., Fosshage, 2013).

However, what is not clear to me in this description of self is how Magid *et al.* think about transference. As described previously, while bi-directional influence is always part of the mix, the patient enters with an organization of self experience that is *not* simply co-created in the analytic relationship. How are we to think and talk about that part? It doesn't seem to me that "preferred ways of being" or stable patterns of attractor states is enough, even though there are aspects of our earlier notions that can be translated into that vocabulary.

There are two reasons I think this matters. One goes to the issue of the inherent asymmetry of the analytic relationship. We can recognize mutuality and reciprocal influence, but, as we know, reciprocal does not mean symmetrical. One person comes seeking help and pays a fee; one person is licensed to provide the help and collects the fee. While both people may be changed by the experience, the *goal* of the relationship is change in one of them, the patient. We can speak about co-transference, but it is the transference of one person that becomes the ultimate focus of their joint efforts. After citing research that has shown that the baby is an initiator and not just a recipient of maternal action, Magid et al. say that the implications of this are controversial in terms of the "meaning and limits of analytic mutuality and nature of asymmetrical responsibility inherent in the analytic relationship" (p. 13). They do not elaborate further on how they define those controversies, limits and responsibilities.

A second, related issue concerns the importance of keeping our focus on the patient's internal, subjective experience. Without being anchored in an ongoing appreciation of this asymmetry, a therapist emphasizing mutual contributions to the analytic couple's joint experience can lead to a focus on what is happening interpersonally and behaviorally between them rather than on the patient's subjective *experience* of those interactions. The unique person the therapist is has an immense impact on what ensues, but not because of what the therapist is or does; rather, it's because of the *meaning* the patient makes of what the therapist does and the internal experience it evokes. For similar reasons, referring to "the selfobject" as a person risks losing its essential meaning as an internal experience.

I have long felt that Donna Orange (1996) articulated this distinction the most helpfully by describing psychoanalytic treatment as the dialogic attempt of two people to examine their joint, co-created experience in order to illuminate (and, I would add, transform) the internal experience of one of them. Orange thus makes explicit a distinction between process and goals. Looking at the experience and contributions of both patient and therapist is a means to an end. There are in fact times when enactments or impasses can only be resolved by a deeper awareness on the part of the therapist about what he or she is bringing to the mix. Particularly strong and helpful illustrations of these phenomena are found in Atwood, Stolorow, and Trop's (1989) description of intersubjective conjunctions and disjunctions. But even there, the goal of the treatment remains the illumination and transformation of the patient's sense of self and self organization.

Because core aspects of the patient's self organization are manifested and/or defended against in the transference, our understanding, attunement and responsiveness to what the patient presents transferentially is a key way we come to understand the nature and state of their self experience. Whatever inadvertent (and inevitable) contributions we make to the process in the room, we do not intentionally try to be something specific. Rather, it is the patient's transference that puts us in the role of a particular kind of other, whether needed or repeated, whether affirming and guiding or critical and rejecting. It is our attention and responsiveness to these overtures that move the treatment forward and facilitate the unfolding of the patient's innate developmental capacities and processes. Another way to say it is that we may be in the same ensemble, but the patient is (and must be) the conductor. Again, recognizing clearly, as Magid et al. do, that the person of the therapist or analyst matters a great deal, there is still just one person in the end whose life we are there to improve, one person whose self we are trying to change, one person who, through our depth of understanding and their new experience with us, we hope will be able to consolidate a freer, more expanded sense of self and a more meaningful and rewarding life.

I believe we can all be grateful to Magid et al. for the mastery, clarity and comprehensiveness with which they have traced the evolution and connections between disparate strands of theory since Kohut's death. I personally found their illumination and integration of the innovations both clarifying and helpful. At the same time, I believe it is important to include a more fulsome description of some continuing core concepts in self psychology, particularly for students and newer clinicians who may be less aware of the through lines from Kohut's original ideas to what we have today.

My hope is that, in their response to the various discussions of their article, Magid *et al.* will also address the questions I've raised here. I have no question that in their practice the authors of Relational Self Psychology thoroughly understand transference and the fact that there is a self that the patient enters with beyond (and before) what is mutually created in the consulting room. But since they do not articulate these things explicitly here, I would like to see them further elaborate their thoughts on the *non-co-created* aspects of transference, the limits of analytic mutuality and the continuities in concepts of self and treatment that they believe continue to guide us. I would look forward to hearing their ideas on these questions.[1]

Note

1 For a response to this chapter and other discussions of their article on relational self psychology by the authors, see Magid, Fosshage, and Shane (2022).

References

Atwood, G., Stolorow, R., & Trop, J. (1989). Impasses in psychoanalytic therapy: A royal road. *Contemporary Psychoanalysis*, *25*, 554–573.

Basch, M. (1988). *Understanding psychotherapy: The science behind the art*. New York, NY: Basic Books.

Beebe, B., & Lachmann, F. (1988). Mother-infant mutual influence and precursors of psychic structure. *Progress in Self Psychology*, *3*, 3–25.

Bowlby, J. (1988). *A secure base*. London, UK: Routledge.

Bruschweiler-Stern, N., Harrison, A.M., Lyons-Ruth, K., Morgan, A.C., Nahum, J.P., Tronick, E.Z., & BCPSG (The Boston Change Process Study Group). (2002). Explicating the implicit: The local level and the microprocess of change in the analytic situation. *The International Journal of Psychoanalysis, 83*, 1051–1062.

Fosshage, J. (2013). Forming and transforming self-experience. *International Journal of Psychoanalytic Self Psychology, 8*, 437–451.

Gardner, J. (2021). Whither the self in relational self psychology? A comment on Magid, Fosshage & Shane's article. *Psychoanalysis, Self and Context, 16*, 315–318.

Kohut, H. (1984). *How does analysis cure*. New York, NY: International Universities Press.

Lyons-Ruth, K. (1999). The two-person unconscious: Intersubjective dialogue, enactive relational representation, and the emergence of new forms of relational organization. *Psychoanalytic Inquiry, 19*, 576–617.

Magid, B., Fosshage, J., & Shane, E. (2021). The emerging paradigm of relational self psychology: A historical perspective. *Psychoanalysis, Self and Context, 16*, 1–23.

Magid, B., Fosshage, J., & Shane, E. (2022). Response to commentaries by Coburn, Gardner and Teicholz on "The emerging paradigm of relational self psychology: An historical perspective." *Psychoanalysis, Self and Context, 17*, 1–7.

Orange, D. (1996, October). *Reconceptualizing the clinical exchange: From the standpoint of intersubjectivity*. Presentation at the 19th Annual Conference on the Psychology of the Self, Washington, DC.

Shane, M., Shane, E., & Gales, M. (1997). *Intimate attachments: Toward a new self-psychology*. New York, NY: Guilford.

Socarides, D., & Stolorow, R. (1984–1985). Affects and selfobjects. *The Annual of Psychoanalysis, 12*, 105–119.

Stern, S. (1994). Needed relationships and repeated relationships an integrated relational perspective. *Psychoanalytic Dialogues, 4*, 317–346.

Stern, S. (2017). *Needed relationships and psychoanalytic healing*. New York, NY: Routledge.

Stolorow, R., Atwood, G., & Brandchaft, B. (1987). *Psychoanalytic treatment: An intersubjective approach*. Hillsdale, NJ: The Analytic Press.

Thelen, E., & Smith, L. (1994). *A dynamic systems approach to the development of cognition and action*. Cambridge, MA: MIT Press.

Tolpin, M. (2002). Doing psychoanalysis of normal development: Forward edge transferences. *Progress in Self Psychology, 18*, 167–190.

Part Three

Chapter 8

Nuances of Empathic Communication

While the role of empathic understanding and responsiveness is central to theories anchored in self psychology and intersubjectivity, appreciating the importance of employing an empathic mode of observation does not necessarily mean that one knows how to do so effectively. The process of achieving and communicating empathic understanding is complex and multiply determined. To help bridge this gap between theory and practice, I offer in this chapter a series of concrete, experience-near suggestions or principles for enhancing empathic understanding and responsiveness. Several writers have stated their belief that empathic resonance is a skill that can be developed through training and learning. I add to those efforts here by defining several choice points and subtleties of how we respond that can make empathic communication more effective. These suggestions emerged from the process of training and supervising mental health professionals in all disciplines and thus are presented as a resource not only for clinicians, but also for teachers and supervisors. This chapter is, in effect, a culmination of what I have gleaned over the past 50+ years about how to help clinicians become more effective in their empathic communication. To create a context and rationale for what follows, the chapter starts with a highly condensed review of our contemporary understanding of the theoretical assumptions that underlie our focus on empathy, including those related to development, psychopathology and therapeutic action.

This paper was published in 2024 as "Forms and Transformations of Empathy: Subtleties and Complexities of Empathic Communication" in Psychoanalysis, Self and Context, *Volume 19.*

My overall goal in this chapter is to link theory and practice about empathy in a concrete, experience-near way by describing some of the practical issues and choices that go into establishing effective empathic understanding and

DOI: 10.4324/9781003491453-11

communication. Embarking on such a project, I think it's important first to answer two questions: 1) Why do we care so much about empathy anyway? and 2) Why do we need yet another article about it? There are three different perspectives from which I'll address these questions and frame what follows.

First, the focus on empathy in self psychology and intersubjectivity theory rests on our particular understanding of development, psychopathology and therapeutic action. So at the outset I will summarize briefly our most relevant underlying theoretical assumptions about these topics in order to clarify the rationale for talking about empathy.

A second context has to do with the broad appeal and utility of these ideas. Although self psychology and intersubjectivity theory emerged originally from the work of psychoanalysts and psychoanalytic researchers, the concepts embodied in these theories have wide applicability to clinicians from all mental health disciplines and practicing in widely varied clinical settings. Our published case studies, however, tilt strongly toward examples of people in psychoanalysis or long-term, intensive psychoanalytic psychotherapy. Before entering full-time private practice, I spent many years working in a hospital-based community mental health center and teaching in a social work school, where people in the students' caseloads included some of the most psychologically, socially, economically and environmentally challenged individuals. In these settings, I have seen how much a deep and effective empathic connection can make a profound difference in people's lives, no matter how briefly offered. Many of the suggestions outlined below emerged from my experience supervising and training mental health professionals in these settings.[1]

This brings me to the third context for writing this article, namely, the challenge of translating theory into practice. As I'll describe below, formulating an empathic response involves a multitude of potential choices at any given moment and is infinitely more complex than any simple prescription to "just say what you hear." One can understand on a theoretical level the rationale for employing an empathic mode of observation and response, but that does not necessarily mean one knows how to do so effectively.

Nevertheless, there is broad consensus that empathic resonance is a skill that can be taught. Kohut (1984) stated that empathy is not a matter of endowment, but rather a product of training and learning. Basch (1988) similarly stated that he believed that empathy was not an inherent talent, but rather something that could be dissected, described, taught and learned.

He outlined a five-step process for reaching empathic understanding. Geist (2013) also took up the challenge of trying to be more explicit about how an analyst or therapist actually enters another's subjective world. Where Basch laid out a series of steps, Geist used the microprocess of a session to formulate and illustrate an intersubjective definition of empathy, emphasizing the mutuality of the process. Goldin (2023) further delineated the empathic process by describing empathy as a dynamic relational process that operates on a continuum from a "what" form of empathy to a "why" or storied form. Finally, Sucharov (2002), emphasizing the thorough embeddedness of empathic understanding in an intersubjective field, suggested that what we do involves less a matter of empathic immersion than what he called an "empathic dance." These are just a few of the previous attempts to delineate how we create empathic responsiveness in the effort to enter the mind of another human being and promote a process of change. The present article strives to add to these efforts.

There is a vast literature on empathy, covering multiple dimensions, its relational meanings and construction, and the dynamics of how it mobilizes growth or "cures." My focus here, however, is narrowly on the concrete and experience-near translation of theory to practice when it comes to *communicating* empathic understanding. There are, similarly, multiple ways to describe and understand the components and process of change in therapy, most of which will also not be addressed here. Rather, I am focusing primarily on just one aspect of therapeutic action, i.e., how the effective communication of empathic understanding enables the identification, elaboration and transformation of the patient's internal experience.

Theoretical Underpinnings

As mentioned above, our focus on empathy rests on assumptions our theory makes about development, psychopathology and therapeutic action. So I'll start with a brief and highly condensed summary of some of the basic assumptions that underlie self psychology and intersubjectivity theory, in order to offer a context for what follows.

In terms of development, we start with the idea that our experience, affects and sense of self are developed and organized (and later reorganized) in specific relational contexts. This means that our early experiences with our primary caregivers lead to ideas about how emotions and relationships work—what's allowed, what's not, what's rewarded, what's punished and so forth. These ideas operate outside of our conscious awareness but powerfully influence our experience and behavior. This patterning has gone by a lot of different names: Organizing principles (Stolorow, Brandchaft, & Attwood, 1987), working models (Bowlby, 1988), patterns of expectation (Beebe & Lachmann, 1988, 1994), emotional convictions (Orange, 1996), implicit relational knowing (BPCSG: Lyons-Ruth, 1999; Stern et al., 1998) or, more recently, attractor states (e.g., Magid, Fosshage, & Shane, 2021; Thelen & Smith, 1994).

When there is a history of chronic misattunement, abuse or developmental trauma, people develop ways of trying to protect against retraumatization. If the environment doesn't lend itself to recognition and acceptance of what is authentically the child's internal experience (volitions, perceptions, etc.), the child will do whatever is necessary to protect the nascent self and the bond with their absolutely needed caregivers. These efforts are manifested in symptoms and defenses, which we understand as adaptations to vulnerability, although their function in these terms may not be obvious initially. When such a person comes into therapy, these adaptations become manifest in their relationship with us as continued attempts to protect the self through methods that have become firmly established for doing so.

A fair amount of therapy involves helping people become aware of and reexamine these implicit assumptions or organizing principles upon which they are conducting their lives. When needed, previous adaptations that are no longer relevant, required or useful need to be modified or transformed in the context of current realities in the patient's life. In therapy, we become a new partner in the patient's affective and relational experience. Through this relationship and a new and different experience with us, a door is opened to the possibility of change in these unconscious patterns.

A major component of treatment, then, involves helping people become aware of and understand their internal experience, what's going on out of their awareness that interferes with them doing, feeling or going after and achieving what they want. This includes affects, needs, adaptations and organizing principles, all these things that may be driving someone's experience and behavior without their realizing it, and much of which will be expressed via the transference, the relationship with us.

When people come into therapy, they do not necessarily begin with this understanding that their own inner processes are playing a major role in creating the experiences that cause them such trouble. Often it is the behavior of others and external forces—whether the unfair boss or work demands, the bully husband, the defiant child or demanding parent—that are presented as the source of their problems, rather than the patient's reactions and response to these people. The unreflected meanings our patients make of their experience and their felt or automatic imperative to accommodate, or withdraw, or defy, or become invisible and so forth constrain their options and paradoxically contribute to the very problems for which they are seeking relief. Much of our work involves bringing these automatic patterns to light, where they can be reexamined. While subjective experience is always contextually and intersubjectively created, the potential for change resides in the patient recognizing and claiming ownership over the part that is internal. This is the part that has the potential to come under their own conscious control and thereby empower them to change their experience, their reactions and their lives.

All this is a very schematic, brief description, but hopefully it is enough to clarify why we put so much emphasis on illuminating and validating the patient's internal reality. But how do we do that, given that we don't have blood tests or scans for internal assumptions or subjective experience? This is where empathy comes in. There are two and only two ways to know about inner life: Introspection is how we can know about our own internal experience, and empathy is how we can know about someone else's. This is why Kohut referred to empathy as vicarious introspection. For him, it was initially an observational stance, one of looking at the world through the eyes of the patient. At the end of his life, Kohut (1981) talked about empathy as therapeutic *per se*, and subsequently just about everyone else has emphasized the therapeutic impact of empathic responsiveness itself. So in our theory we focus on subjective experience, because that is the point of entry to the patient's inner life, and we focus on empathy because that is the *means* by which we gain access to that inner world.

Complexity of Formulating an Empathic Response

What do we have to do to establish empathic contact with our patient? We could say, "Just say what you hear or understand, without adding, subtracting, or redirecting it." But already then we're going to be lost. If I want to go from New York to California and I'm told, "Just go west," I suppose I might eventually get there, but certainly not efficiently, and I'm likely to be clueless about where to turn next at many junctures. Also, *how* should I say what I hear and which part of it? Is it better to use the patient's words or my own? Should I reflect feelings or behavior? Results or intentions? Events or reactions? Hopes or fears? Forward edge or trailing? These are all moment-by-moment decision points and choices. What about my tone of voice and non-verbal behavior? And complicating all of this is the fact that whatever we hear and potentially convey back to our patients is filtered through our own lenses and organizing principles. As Stolorow is fond of putting it, there is no immaculate perception. Our own history and organizing principles will impact both our expectations and our perceptions of what we've heard.

Since empathy *per se* is value neutral, we constantly make choices about how to use our empathic understanding to respond in ways that facilitate and advance the treatment process. So in what follows I'd like to offer some suggestions or possibilities regarding what to attend to or focus on in order to do the following: 1) Achieve an accurate empathic understanding; 2) Communicate that understanding in a way that enables the patient to *feel* deeply understood; 3) Advance the therapeutic process by promoting the unfolding of the patient's interior life; and 4) Provide a new relational experience. These are all among the central functions of empathy. I've organized my suggestions under seven subheadings, illustrated with brief examples, and then followed by two additional vignettes that reflect a combination of the various interventions I've described.

Affect and Underlying Needs, Wishes or Intentions

As I said earlier, our affective experience becomes organized and reorganized in specific relational contexts. For many of our patients, the therapist's affective attunement provides a developmentally missing and corrective experience, which helps people both identify and feel the validity or legitimacy of their feelings. Kohut actually described the therapist's affective responsiveness as being at the heart of what is curative in treatment. So we naturally emphasize the patient's feelings, first and foremost, in our empathic reflections. But when, in addition to reflecting reactive affects, we also reflect the patient's underlying wishes, we belatedly legitimize selfobject needs that have been previously thwarted.

For example, with a patient who was upset with her family for being totally focused on their usual arguments with each other when they went out to dinner after her graduation rather than celebrating her achievement, the therapist not only reflected her hurt, disappointment and anger, but also said, "What you wanted was for them to be proud of you, to be able to set all that aside and pay attention to *you* for once, on your special day." To another patient whose AA sponsor gave her a lecture when she slipped and had a drink, the therapist said, "You felt criticized when you hoped for support." These kinds of responses not only help the patient feel deeply understood; they also help them undo the disavowal of needs that have been sequestered due to misattunement in the past. It is only when people feel the legitimacy of their needs that they can take actions to express and get them met. For the graduate, it was a response to her need for mirroring/affirmation; for the recovering alcoholic, a response to her need for idealized strength and guidance.

This also relates to fostering a sense of personal agency. Agency refers to the capacity to act effectively on one's own initiative, being in the driver's seat of one's own life. Hagman (2020) has written that promoting a sense of personal agency involves more than affect attunement. We also need to be empathic to the child as a center of initiative and action. Parents do this by naming and organizing the child's intentions. For example, sitting with a young child playing with blocks, a parent might say, "You're piling the blocks so high; you're making something very tall, maybe like a tower?" i.e., the parent is echoing not just how the experience feels (it's fun to play with blocks), but what the child is trying to *do*. I am suggesting that when we start to convey our empathic understanding to our patients, in addition to reflecting their affect there is therapeutic mileage to be gained from also listening for, naming and affirming the patient's underlying needs, wishes, longings and/or intentions.

Focusing on What is Present not Absent

A child wants her mother to go with her into the therapist's office. Rather than saying, "You're not willing to go into the office by yourself" or even "Why do you want your mother there?" it's more useful to say, "You must have a (good) reason for wanting your mother there." In other words, we focus on what she is doing (wanting mother) rather than what she is not doing (going in alone). With someone who constantly jumps the gun, so to speak, reacting too quickly or impulsively, rather than suggesting, "You need to be more patient," we'd want to say, "It's hard to be patient." In other words, we stay with the patient's actual experience and say what we hear, rather than doing something else or trying to get them to do something else.

Another patient complained that his wife was constantly intruding on his Zoom therapy sessions, which he didn't like or want. In a presumably well-meaning effort to legitimize the patient's desires, the therapist wanted to urge him to push back against his wife's intrusion into his treatment. But I'm suggesting that we would want instead to explore his *not* doing so; e.g., "I gather that even though you don't like it, you don't feel you can tell her to stop." This shifts the focus from his behavior to whatever internal experience is driving it. When we are using empathic responsiveness to connect with and elaborate internal experience, we need to focus on what is already present and available to the patient, aiming to expand *that* rather than directing the patient's attention elsewhere. This is what we mean when we talk about empathic immersion and staying experience near.

Specific Meanings of Word Choice

What a word means to us may be very different from what the same word means to our patient. I say to my patient, "You don't feel entitled to have what you want." She says, "No, John (her husband) is entitled; it's more like I don't deserve it." To me, it feels pretty equivalent or synonymous to say someone doesn't feel entitled to something or doesn't feel they deserve it, but not to her. That did not make her feel understood. In the correction, she clarifies that she doesn't feel she deserves something different because she feels she has enabled his behavior, contributed to creating this situation by her passivity and therefore forfeited her right to have what she wants, i.e., to deserve it.

The Ornsteins (P. Ornstein & Ornstein, 1985) also had a wonderful example of this in an early paper in which the therapist commented on how the patient's dream reflected how he had been rescued from a dangerous situation. The patient felt deeply hurt and misunderstood, because he felt he had *escaped* from the situation by dint of his own strength and resourcefulness. He wanted the therapist to appreciate this. Saying he was rescued made him feel instead that the therapist saw him as passive and dependent, rather than strong and resourceful.

It's also worth thinking about the way specific words carry an emotional punch. Two examples in English I've found particularly vivid and resonant for patients are the words "stranded" and "ambushed." Interestingly, each implies both an action by an outside force or person and an internal response to it, thereby condensing a great deal into just one word. Others reading this have probably found other specific words to be particularly powerful in capturing their patients' experiences.

Efforts at empathic immersion help us locate the right word or words to capture the patient's experience. But as we talk about the importance of what meanings specific words have for the patient, it is important to remember that we don't have to be, and often can't be, immediately right. We have to be flexible, meaning we have to let the patient correct us when we get it wrong. Only the patient can determine whether they feel understood, and until someone feels we understand how it is for them, they can't make use of anything else we might say, no matter how "true" we might think it is.

External Triggers, Internal Experience and Sequence

People often describe their experience in terms of something they or someone else did and their reaction to it. In responding, it's helpful to emphasize or describe the internal experience more than the external trigger. Consider these two statements: "They didn't believe you" *vs* "You felt discounted by them." These describe the same event and seem to mean roughly the same thing, but one is talking about them, the other, and one about you, the patient. One describes behavior, the other describes affect.

A related point concerns the sequence in which we say things. People tend to elaborate from the place we end. So, when possible, it's helpful to emphasize and end with the part we hope to expand. Consider a situation where someone is at a bar with friends and then the others move on to the next bar without saying when or where. We could say, "You felt deserted when all the others left without you," or "When all the others left without you, you felt deserted." The sentences mean the same thing and even have exactly the same words, but the first may be more likely to evoke an elaboration of how the others left (their behavior), while the second pulls more for an elaboration of the deserted feelings, the internal experience. This distinction may sound like splitting hairs and less relevant in a short sentence like this, but can become more important when responding to a long description of an event and its impact on the patient.

Tone and Other Non-verbal Aspects of Our Words

The same word can convey a wide range of different meanings depending on the tone with which it is uttered. If I say, in a flat voice, "That made you furious," the empathic impact is going to be a lot different than if I say, "That made you FURIOUS!" Our body posture, our sighs, our leaning in or back and other gestures all communicate aspects of understanding. Sometimes we convey our empathic response in ways that don't use or paraphrase the patient's words at all. In response to one patient who described to me someone's outrageous and exasperating behavior, I blurted out, with considerable emphasis and no forethought, "Oh, for God's sake!" She stopped, let out a big sigh and simply said, "Thank you," signaling clearly to me that she felt totally understood. I'm reminded here of Kohut's patient with whom he simply synchronized his breathing to convey an empathic connection (Kohut, 1984).[2]

Intersubjective Conjunction and Disjunction

These terms refer to ways that the organizing patterns and defenses of the two people in the therapeutic dyad intersect and co-create particular outcomes. Both reflect the interaction of their separately organized subjective worlds. How *we* see the world may be similar to or different from how our patient does. Those differences include not only our perceptions, but also our expectations, our reactions, our needs and values and, importantly, our own defenses. As Atwood, Stolorow, and Trop (1989) have described, places where patient and therapist view the world the same way (i.e., intersubjective conjunctions) may be seen as reflections of objective reality rather than manifestations of the patient's personality. When a defensive solution is shared by patient and therapist, they note that it may escape analytic inquiry and/or put them at odds with each other. Such conjunctions may result in empathic ruptures/derailments or in mutual strengthening of resistance that may prolong the treatment.

Here's one of their examples, in brief. A patient complained about the impossibility of finding meaningful attachments because of the mechanization and depersonalization of modern life, a view of society that the therapist happened to share. So, seeing the patient's attitude as a reflection of objective reality rather than manifestations of his conflictual issues concerning intimacy and attachment, those issues were never explored. This example and several others can be found in the authors' article on impasses in psychoanalytic treatment (Atwood et al., 1989).

What we hear in our patients can be limited by what we can hear (or stand to hear) in ourselves. So these intersubjective conjunctions and disjunctions create potential impediments to empathic immersion and understanding. For this reason, accurate empathic understanding often necessitates that therapists become reflectively aware of the principles that govern our own internal experience.

In the decades since Atwood et al. wrote about these ideas, the literature in self psychology and intersubjectivity theory has shifted toward an even more thoroughgoing emphasis on bi-directionality, mutual impact and co-creation of experience in the analytic relationship. While I do not further elaborate on this focus in the present chapter, it is important to underscore how much these phenomena impact the process of empathic understanding. It is decisively important not only who the patient is, but who the listening therapist or analyst is. For those who seek a deeper understanding of this dimension of the process, a good place to start includes the articles mentioned earlier by Geist (2013) and Sucharov (2002), as well as Perlitz's (2022) work on mutual embeddedness.

Forward Edge and Trailing Edge

One of the most important and useful concepts we have for guiding our empathic listening and response is the concept of the forward edge. This term came from Kohut, was described initially in an article by Jule Miller (1985) and was then later elaborated by Marian Tolpin (2002) and others.

By way of definition, forward edge refers to transference and/or other expressions of thwarted but still remaining healthy, childhood, developmental needs. Trailing edge refers to transference and/or other expressions of repetitive patterns, negative expectations and defensive strategies which have developed as a result of trauma, misattunement and empathic failure. So trailing edge comments address what the patient is trying to defend against, deny or ward off. Forward edge interpretations address the patient's strivings and hopes. Frank Lachmann (2016) noted that forward edge interpretations speak to "what the patient is trying to attain, retain or maintain through symptoms and behaviors that may look like pathology" to the observer, but actually reflect the patient's motivational strivings (p. 501).

In describing the importance of this concept, Marian Tolpin (2002) emphasized that accepting whatever tendrils of healthy self there are and addressing that forward edge of health are what provide the motive force for resumed development in therapy. She also believed that an accurate understanding of the forward edge, as experienced in the treatment relationship, constituted the seeding of a new experience. This, of course, is very consistent with what I said earlier about the therapist as a new affective partner, with whom new, co-created experiences can begin to transform the patient's expectations and internal world.

By way of example, Jule Miller, who was in supervision with Kohut, told him about a patient who Miller thought wanted to avoid his inner life by picking a fight with him. Kohut suggested instead commenting to the patient that picking fights was a way he had kept himself from feeling empty over the years and of making meaningful contact with the people important to him. It's a really nice example of how, even in the context of what is undoubtedly a very problematic relational pattern of provoking others, this kind of understanding and comment on the healthy wish to make meaningful contact with others helps nurture that striving. It's what Marian Tolpin (2002) called "blowing on the embers." This not only sets the stage for the emergence of a more full-blown selfobject transference but, ultimately, helps him find less costly and more fulfilling ways of meaningful engagement with others.[3]

Here's another example, this one from the same paper on agency by Hagman (2020) I mentioned earlier. Hagman described a patient, David, who effectively shut him out during sessions by insisting on "doing his own analysis." A trailing edge interpretation might see this as resistance and defensive self-sufficiency. Hagman instead interpreted this as an attempt to avoid coercive intrusion by the therapist that would usurp his authentic experience, a feared repetition of his chronic history with his mother. So protecting and preserving his authentic sense of self was the forward edge here.

As I said above, when talking about what's present versus what's absent, it's important for us to place our emphasis on what our patients are striving to do rather than what they are trying to avoid and what is right, i.e., healthy, about their choices rather than what is wrong or pathological. Hagman's forward edge understanding and interpretation of David needing initially to shut him out not only enables his patient to feel understood in depth, it offers belated recognition and affirmation of his creative act of self-preservation. Importantly, this facilitates his dawning awareness of his own role in authoring the actions that now cause him great difficulty.

Because our patients generally start out with no awareness of these dynamics and phenomena, the things that on a deep level propel their behavior and inform and constrict their experience, it is imperative to stay initially with what is consciously available and not prematurely threaten what has been the patient's best or only way of protecting themselves. This is what empathic immersion and staying focused on the forward edge enable and lead us to do. When Hagman does this by restraining his own desire to interpret and allowing David to keep him shut out, he cultivates an environment of trust and safety, free of the threat of coercion or impingement. The goal is to enable David, and all such patients, eventually to see that their difficulties are not a product of external forces, but rather of internal choices made long ago that have become rigid and constraining. It is the sustained empathic immersion in our patients' internal worlds that allows us to bring about this result.[4]

Here's a last illustration, this one an example of how the concept of the forward edge reorients my empathic listening. At the end of a first session, my patient asks if he can pay in advance for his sessions. Some people don't like to write a check every week or get a big bill at the end of the month, so I tell him that would be fine. He writes a check and leaves it on my desk. After he leaves, I look at the check and see that it is for $5,000. I wonder various things: Is he trying to impress me? compete with me? counteract the humiliation of coming for help by being a big man and throwing his money around? But listening for the forward edge, when he returns I simply note the size of the check and invite his thoughts about it. It turns out that he was someone who had tried therapy many times in the past, but would always blow it off or drop out. The large check, covering many months of sessions, was a way of trying to secure a commitment from himself to stay in treatment.

What people do is nearly always in the service of protecting the self (their agency, vitality, autonomy) or protecting a bond with a needed other. Listening for these things with that orientation makes a profound difference in what we hear and how we respond. To find the forward edge, it helps to start with the assumption that there is something right in what the patient is doing and to listen for how. When we see symptoms or seemingly dysfunctional behavior, it can help to ask ourselves the question, "To what problem is this behavior a solution?" (What could conceivably make *me* do what this person is doing?) Seeking the answer can help clarify internal dynamics and forward edge motivations. In my last example, the large check was an attempted solution to the problem of fleeing from therapy before giving it a chance to help.

Illustrative Vignettes

I've been describing under these various subheadings things that I see as relevant to enhancing effective empathic communication and responsiveness, all in the service of achieving our therapeutic aims—the resolution of presenting problems, resumed development, increased sense of agency and so forth. I'd like to finish with two brief vignettes which capture many of the ideas I've described.

Vignette #1

My patient is 33, single, and longing to find a suitable marriage partner with whom she can settle down and build a life. She is having an intense affair with a man who lives a thousand miles away and is married with two young children, a family he has no interest in leaving. He is very jealous and possessive toward my patient, particularly grilling her if she pays any attention to other men. For the zillionth time we are discussing what draws her into and sustains this relationship. She says, "He challenges me, he probes and pushes me to say things I don't want to say, things that are hard. Like when I had dinner with Sam [a former boyfriend], he wanted to know if we had sex and he kept pushing. I told him it was none of his business. But he doesn't let up. It's hard for me to answer because I feel guilty, but he forces me to be honest. It's good for me. I can't hide from him."

At this point, I'm trying to keep my bearings, because what I feel like doing is screaming at her, "What are you talking about? This man is married and almost completely unavailable, yet he suggests that *you* are cheating if you hook up with an old boyfriend? And this is what you consider helping you grow by forcing you to look at yourself and be honest?" I feel like Dr. Phil and want to say, "Get real!"

But then I remember Kohut's (1984) famous dictum that the patient's rightness is likely to be more profound than his, so I refocus, give it another try and say to her, "There's something about being able to tell him things that are hard to say, that he won't like hearing—that feels very important to you." She replies, "Yes, all my life I've had to hide who I really am. I can never show my parents what's really going on. They would be so disappointed. But Jake just accepts me." I finally start to get it. "So it's in the way he accepts you *after* you've leveled with him about something he won't like that you finally feel you can be who you really are." She starts to cry (signaling we've hit an affective nerve) and says, "Yes, I feel like I've been hiding my whole life. It's the only place I can be honest." I reply, "It's such a relief to feel at last you can be yourself, not have to hide, and still feel worthwhile. Finally you can feel loveable and loved for who you are, rather than who you think others need you to be. That just feels so great." She cries harder.

Then she says, "I remember the first time I deliberately hid something from my parents. I lied to do it. It still haunts me." She then elaborated the incident in some detail and how it left her wracked with shame and guilt. The central importance of hiding, secrets, guilt and shame were coming into sharper relief and beginning to shed light on my patient's dynamics and struggles.

By reorienting myself to the importance of empathic immersion and the forward edge, I was able to transform my negative feelings into an empathic response which facilitated an unfolding clinical process. Following Kohut's dictum (that the patient is always right somehow, listen for it) made possible an empathic response which yielded an upsurge of affect, a confirming association/story and an expansion of the thematic content so important to understanding the dynamics of what was keeping my patient in this ultimately unfulfilling affair. This vignette is an illustration of what I meant before when I said we are trying to use the empathic process to illuminate and promote an unfolding of the patient's internal experience.

Vignette #2

This next vignette is from a supervision session with a therapist who comes for consultation on her private practice cases. I chose it because of the ways it illustrates a process and attitude I'm trying to convey.

My supervisee says, apologetically and somewhat shamefully, that she runs over the time with one of her patients and doesn't end the sessions on time. She says, "I know this is wrong, I shouldn't be doing it" in a way that feels to me almost like a little kid confessing that she got into the cookie jar and ate all the cookies, i.e., I'm bad.

So my first step is to create a different context and framework for looking at this, moving from condemnation to exploration, a process not that different from how we try to engage our patients. To create a safer space for her to explore the situation, I suggest that we shift from the idea that "you're doing something wrong" to the idea that "you're doing something for reasons you don't yet understand." In concert with what I described earlier as addressing what's present rather than absent, the focus is not on what she's *not* doing (ending on time), but on what she *is* doing (running over time).

We proceed as follows: I ask if she generally runs over with patients. She says, "No." I say, "So there must be a reason for it with this person." She replies, "I feel I have to give the person more time." Why is that? She reports, "I withdraw toward the end of the session."

I ask if she could elaborate and I encourage her associations. She says, "This patient has very poor boundaries; I feel like I could get engulfed by her."

Continuing the exploration along these lines, the dynamics become more clear. It turns out the therapist gets more quiet and withdrawn about 10 minutes before the end of the session as a response to her experience of her patient as "too needy" (her words) and potentially engulfing. Eventually she realizes she's checked out and feels guilty about having withdrawn from her patient, and so she offers her extra time to compensate, which leads to running over time.

Like our patients, she doesn't start out knowing all this. She just comes in confessing that she's doing something wrong. She needs help to identify what's going on internally that's driving this behavior. What enables me to help her is my attitude, my way of thinking about things, by maintaining an empathic focus and searching for the positive (and initially hidden) function of her behavior. (Cf. what problem is this behavior a solution to?)

This requires an open minded, non-judgmental curiosity, as well as an initial tolerance for uncertainty and ambiguity, for not knowing. As my own mentor, Miriam Elson (personal communication), often said, "The tolerance for ambiguity is the hallmark of a professional." This becomes much easier when we hold a firm belief that empathy will enable us to find out what we (and they) don't yet know. Self psychology and intersubjectivity theory, especially concepts like empathic immersion and the forward edge, help us to understand and cultivate this kind of attitude.

Conclusion

These ideas about nuances of empathic communication help me to be effective, and my hope is that writing about them will similarly help others be ever more effective in their own work. Empathic understanding and responsiveness aren't easy, automatic or simple, but nothing is more powerful in revealing our patients' internal worlds, offering them a new experience and helping them change their lives.

Notes

1 More detailed reports of the use of self psychology theory in short-term treatment can be found in chapters 2 and 3 of this volume (also Gardner (1991, 1999).
2 Descriptions of additional procedures by which other authors have described how non-verbal expressions, bodily sensations and posture can facilitate empathic understanding and communication can be found in the work of Brothers and Sletvold (2022, 2023) and Nebbiosi and Federici (2022).
3 At the time Miller's article was published, homosexuality was still considered pathological and was included as a diagnosis in the DSM. There has been considerable criticism of Miller's understanding and treatment of homosexuality from our contemporary perspective. Nevertheless, I believe that much of his article remains valuable for its informative examples of how Kohut understood the concept of responding to the forward edge. For a contemporary perspective on the homoerotic aspects of Jule Miller's case, see Sandmeyer (2019).
4 An extended discussion of this case can be found in chapter 6.

References

Atwood, G., Stolorow, R., & Trop, J. (1989). Impasses in psychoanalytic therapy: A royal road. *Contemporary Psychoanalysis, 25*, 554–573.

Basch, M. (1988). *Understanding psychotherapy*. New York, NY: Basic Books.

Beebe, B., & Lachmann, F. (1988). Mother-infant mutual influence and precursors of psychic structure. In A. Goldberg (Ed.), *Progress in self psychology* (Vol. 3, pp. 3–26). Hillsdale, NJ: Analytic Press.

Beebe, B., & Lachmann, F. (1994). Representation and internalization in infancy: Three principles of salience. *Psychoanalytic Psychology, 11*, 127–165.

Bowlby, J. (1988). *A secure base*. London, UK: Routledge.

Brothers, D., & Sletvold, J. (2022). Talking bodies: A new vision of psychoanalysis. *Psychoanalytic Inquiry, 42*, 289–302.

Brothers, D., & Sletvold, J. (2023). *A new vision of psychoanalytic theory, practice and supervision: Talking bodies*. New York, NY: Routledge.

Gardner, J. (1991). The application of self psychology to brief psychotherapy. *Psychoanalytic Psychology, 8*, 477–500.

Gardner, J. (1999). Using self psychology in brief psychotherapy. *Psychoanalytic Social Work, 6*, 43–85.

Gardner, J. (2020). Discussion of George Hagman's "Self-agency: Freedom and context in psychoanalysis." *Psychoanalysis, Self and Context, 15*, 40–46.

Gardner, J. (2024). Forms and transformations of empathy: Subtleties and complexities of empathic communication. *Psychoanalysis, Self and Context, 19*, 80–93.

Geist, R.A. (2013). How the empathic process heals: A microprocess perspective. *International Journal of Psychoanalytic Self Psychology, 8*, 265–281.

Goldin, D. (2023, October). *Empathy on a continuum.* Paper presented at the 44th Annual Conference, International Association for Psychoanalytic Self Psychology, Chicago, IL.

Hagman, G. (2020). Self-agency: Freedom and context in psychoanalysis. *Psychoanalysis, Self and Context, 15*, 33–39.

Kohut, H. (1981). On empathy. In P. Ornstein (Ed.), *The search for the self: Selected writings of Heinz Kohut* (Vol. 4, pp. 525–535). Madison, CT: International Universities Press.

Kohut, H. (1984). *How does analysis cure?* Chicago, IL: University of Chicago Press.

Lachmann, F. (2016). Credo. *Psychoanalytic Dialogues, 26*, 499–512.

Lyons-Ruth, K. (1999). The two-person unconscious: Intersubjective dialogue, enactive relational representation, and the emergence of new forms of relational organization. *Psychoanalytic Inquiry, 19*, 576–617.

Magid, B., Fosshage, J., & Shane, E. (2021). The emerging paradigm of relational self psychology: A historical perspective. *Psychoanalysis, Self and Context, 16*, 1–23.

Miller, J. (1985). How Kohut actually worked. In A. Goldberg (Ed.), *Progress in self psychology* (Vol. 1, pp. 13–30). New York, NY: The Guilford Press.

Nebbiosi, G., & Federici, S. (2022). Miming and clinical psychoanalysis: Enhancing our intersubjective sensibility. *Psychoanalytic Inquiry, 42*, 266–277.

Orange, D. (1996, October). *Reconceptualizing the clinical exchange: From the standpoint of intersubjectivity.* Paper presented at the 19th Annual Conference on the Psychology of the Self, Washington, DC.

Ornstein, P., & Ornstein, A. (1985). Clinical understanding and explaining: The empathic vantage point. In A. Goldberg (Ed.), *Progress in self psychology* (Vol. 1, pp. 43–61). New York, NY: The Guilford Press.

Perlitz, D. (2022). Mutual embeddedness: The foundation for a relational world. *Psychoanalysis, Self and Context, 17*, 8–22.

Sandmeyer, J. (2019). Understanding homophobia in our forefathers: Rethinking how Kohut actually worked. *Psychoanalysis, Self and Context, 14*, 376–392.

Stern, D., Sander, L., Nahum, J., Harriso, A., Lyons-Ruth, K., Morgan, A., Bruschweilerstern, N., & Tronick, E. (1998). Non-interpretive mechanisms in psychoanalytic therapy: The "something more" than interpretation. *International Journal of Psychoanalysis, 79*, 903–921.

Stolorow, R., Brandchaft, B., & Atwood, G. (1987). *Psychoanalytic treatment: An intersubjective approach.* Hillsdale, NJ: The Analytic Press.

Sucharov, M. (2002). Representation and the intrapsychic: Cartesian barriers to empathic contact. *Psychoanalytic Inquiry, 22*, 686–707.

Thelen, E., & Smith, L. (1994). *A dynamic systems approach to the development of cognition and action.* Hillsdale, NJ: The Analytic Press.

Tolpin, M. (2002). Doing psychoanalysis of normal development: Forward edge transferences. In A. Goldberg (Ed.), *Progress in self psychology* (Vol. 18, pp. 167–190). Hillsdale, NJ: The Analytic Press.

Chapter 9

Self Psychology

Journeys and Generations

I chose to end this book with the Kohut lecture I gave in Jerusalem in 2014, as a retrospective summary of my journey toward becoming a self psychologist. Believing that becoming a competent practitioner requires both didactic and experiential learning, I note four vectors for such learning: reading, meetings, mentors and personal therapy. My experiences of transformative moments in each of these areas are described, and I encourage readers to reflect on analogous experiences in their own professional development. Consistent with the theme that runs throughout the chapters of this book, the reader will note that all the examples of my own transformative moments have the experience-near quality I have been emphasizing throughout. I also underscore in this chapter the importance of cross-fertilization across generations by encouraging younger clinicians to reach out to more senior people and more experienced clinicians to actively help nurture and develop the next generation of self psychologists. Vehicles for doing so are described.

This paper was published in 2015 as "Journeys and Generations: Tending the Professional Self" in Psychoanalysis, Self and Context, *Volume 10.*

I would like to dedicate these remarks to the memory of my mentor, Miriam Elson, without whom I surely would not have been able to write this piece. I recognize the fact that being asked to give the Kohut Memorial Lecture is quite an honor. So I want to thank those who invited me to give the talk, as well as create this version for publication, and express my deep appreciation for both the honor and the vote of confidence it expresses.

Having attended my first self psychology conference in 1987, I have heard 25 Kohut Memorial Lectures. Some have wonderfully entertained me, like when Frank Lachmann played excerpts from his beloved operas. Some have moved me. I don't know that I will ever hear a Kohut Memorial

DOI: 10.4324/9781003491453-12

Lecture as incredibly moving as the one given by Donna Orange in 2007. Some, frankly, have bored me. The authors of those, of course, will remain nameless, but the problem was a talk simply too heavy and dense to process on a full stomach.[1] And there is the one I remember the best, ironically one of the earliest I heard, given by Paul Ornstein in Washington, DC, in 1988.

Ornstein was addressing the draw of Kohut's ideas and why he thought they would endure. Contrasting them with other popular, contemporary theories of narcissism and the self, Paul described how with other theories people would tell him that the descriptions and ideas spoke to their practice and taught them about their patients. About reactions to Kohut's work, they told him, "Kohut speaks to *me* ... I can see myself in all of this ... it must be true ... it is certainly true of me." He felt that our need to make self-reflective contact with our own disturbing emotional experiences would always draw us strongly to an approach that promised such an understanding. I think it is also for this reason that the ideas embodied in self psychology are so personally compelling to so many people who read them. We see ourselves in it, and it is, after all, through our own subjective experience that we find our most cherished beliefs—and our theoretical home.

So, how *do* you keep the attention of an audience after a full meal? Well, like most things in self psychology, I figured it starts with empathy—in Jerusalem, empathy with the listeners, and now, with you the reader. I think that means: Say something relevant; try to be at least a little funny if you can, or at least interesting, if you can; don't make it too long; and don't wander all over the place and get everyone lost. So, in the interest of the latter, I'll offer a roadmap for where I'm going by saying how I came up with this title: "Journeys and Generations: Tending the Professional Self."

The phrase "tending the professional self" comes from the title of an article I wrote on supervision (Gardner, 1995). There, I emphasized the needs and vulnerabilities of the learning therapist, themes that I will highlight in this article.

As for journeys, my point of reference and departure is the book of Genesis. In the Jewish calendar of readings from the Torah at the time I delivered my Kohut Lecture, we were coming to a portion of Genesis that is called "*Lech Lecha*." These are Hebrew words that God spoke to Abraham, literally meaning to go forth. Abraham is to leave his home in Ur, the text says, and go "to the place (or land) that I will show you." I've written about these verses a few times in a different context, and to me the heart of it is about journeys. It's about change, going into the unknown, with the promise or hope of getting to a better place. Sounds a lot like psychotherapy.

I often think about *Lech Lecha* in the fall of the year and how to make it relevant to my life in the present.

So, since it's about journeys, I chose in my Kohut Lecture to describe the professional journey to becoming a self psychologist, the journey from student, novice, intern or candidate, through experienced clinician, to supervisor, teacher, mentor and author. Some of us go through all those stops along the way, some through only a portion of them. I want to describe *my* journey, highlight the aspects of it that I think are crucial for anyone wanting to be a self psychologist and encourage you to think about and reflect on your own professional journeys.

Finally (still explaining my title), what about generations? When I wondered whether I had enough to say to accept the invitation to give the Kohut Lecture, my colleague, Brenda Solomon, encouraged me to do so by noting that most of Kohut's original collaborators had spoken, most were physicians and analysts, and I represented something different, "the next generation." This got me thinking about generations. Who are my ancestors, professionally speaking? What was passed on to me by the people who came before? What can I pass along to the people who come after? Depending on where you are in your own trajectory, how can you find the people and experiences you need to grow professionally? How can you give back by nurturing and helping the next generation of self psychologists? What do they need from you and what can you offer to them?

Self psychology was born in the context of psychoanalysis, and I believe that there may be nothing that compares to the depth and richness of psychoanalytic training. Under the dedicated leadership of Roger Segalla and Chuck Finlon, the International Association for Psychoanalytic Self Psychology (IAPSP) has striven to link candidates and institutes around the world and increase their inclusion of self psychological ideas in their curricula. This is a wonderful and important development.

At the same time, there are many people who are deeply immersed and interested in these theories, but have not been and never will be formally trained as psychoanalysts. I am one such person. Our members come from the fields of social work, psychology, counseling, medicine and nursing; they work in the diverse settings of clinics, schools, hospitals and social service organizations, along with private practice; they serve some of the most economically and socially disadvantaged populations; and they find self psychology deeply helpful and relevant for their work. I want to speak for and to all of us, whatever our discipline, training or area of practice.

In 1973, I was given a copy of Kohut's *Analysis of the Self* (Kohut, 1971) as a gift. I could not understand a word of it. In 2014, 41 years later, I found myself invited to give a Kohut Memorial Lecture. How did this happen? What was *my* path and how can describing it help you define and make choices about your own paths, again whether you are new to this or a seasoned clinician and contributor to our field? I recognize that people reading these words may be on a wide swath of this continuum, from beginning students to our most prolific and esteemed writers and teachers.

Just as all psychoanalytic theory incorporates and draws on Freud's seminal ideas but has modified, expanded and gone far beyond them, I believe in the realm of self psychology we all continue to draw on Kohut's seminal, radical-for-his-time innovations, but similarly have since modified, expanded and gone beyond them. The list is too long and probably unnecessary to recite here, but to name even a few, infant research, intersubjectivity theory, neuroscience and so much more now inform our self psychology theories and practice.

When I reflect on my journey through my training and all these subsequent developments, I realize there are four strands that, woven together, created the fabric of who I've become professionally: readings, meetings, mentors and personal therapy. In each arena there were for me heightened affective moments (Beebe & Lachmann, 1994) and transformative experiences. I want to describe some of those to you. And, given that I think these four strands are relevant to all of us, my hope is that my describing this will stimulate you to think about what your own version of it is. What did you read that changed your thinking? Whom did you hear that moved you deeply? Who took an interest in your professional development and helped you have faith and confidence in yourself? And, after perhaps a long personal therapy or analysis, what specific moments or experiences transformed you and remain, even years later, vividly remembered? These are the things I want us to think about.

For me, all four strands came together starting in 1987. Before then, though already working in the field for 14 years, I had had little exposure to self psychology. That year I started therapy (and later analysis) with Paul Tolpin,[2] I attended my first international self psychology conference, I reconnected with Miriam Elson, who was to become my mentor, and I read Miriam's book *Self Psychology in Clinical Social Work* (Elson, 1986), which was the first thing I read in self psychology that I could understand.

I had known Miriam briefly during graduate school, several years earlier, and our paths crossed occasionally after that. But at that first conference I ran into her at the Kohut Lecture lunch and she said, "It's so nice to see you in all the right places!" After that we forged a deeper relationship and she became my mentor.

The need for mentors is described by Brightman (1984) in an article which highlights the narcissistic vulnerability of therapists in training. Brightman describes student aspirations as initially reflecting a triad of idealized attributes that determine professional self-esteem. These are omniscience, benevolence and omnipotence, an image of oneself as the all-knowing, all-loving, all-powerful therapist. As soon as people actually start doing clinical work, they are confronted with the unrealistic aspects of this image. As the real and idealized versions of their professional self-image inevitably collide, they face the threat of narcissistic injury and a precipitous loss of self-esteem.

To manage the tension generated by this struggle between the demands of clinical training, their novice level of skill and their perfectionistic aspirations, students need the support of an idealized mentor who can provide a holding environment (Winnicott, 1965) in which they can modify their professional self-image to something more moderate and attainable. Then, Brightman explains, as the trainee's belief in his or her professional worth grows, the need to be part of someone else's competence diminishes and a gradual de-idealization process occurs.

Miriam Elson was the perfect embodiment of what Brightman was talking about. She understood with tremendous depth the vulnerabilities and strivings of the learner. She had an ability to hold people in their state of not knowing and affirm their fledgling attempts at mastery, along with a remarkable capacity to find the kernel of health or strength in anything, no matter how hidden or obscure. In that way, she showed me a new way of looking at the world. Miriam was also endlessly calm, kind and affirming. She was unstinting in her efforts to nurture the potential of others and their own contributions to our field, encouraging all of us to write or teach. By doing and being all this, she helped build in others a sense of their own competence and confidence. As a result of her guidance, encouragement and support, I began to teach and to write in the area of self psychology. Largely due to her example, I also learned what the people I was training really needed from me.

Initially using the bibliography in Miriam's book as a guide, I started reading other works in self psychology—seminal papers by Marian Tolpin and Michael Basch, the still amazing article entitled "Affects and

Selfobjects" by Socarides and Stolorow (1984–1985), then Ernie Wolf's beautiful *Treating the Self* (1988) and, eventually, even Kohut (1977, 1984) in the original, this time able to understand it.

I want to share briefly some ideas from a few of the articles I read during those early days that simply changed me. The first included the following vignette, written by Arnold Goldberg. The patient told his analyst at a Monday session that he had spent much of the previous weekend at public men's rooms, voyeuristically "peeking" at the other men while they urinated. In the therapist's words,

> He reported a sense of feeling bizarre. In a desolate voice, he reported having spent the times he was not in men's rooms painting empty chairs in his apartment. Suddenly he shouted, "I demand to know what you are thinking. You think I'm psychotic don't you?" The therapist replied, "I think you must have been very lonely." There was a pause, and then [the patient] burst out crying. When he was able to speak again, he said in a choked voice, "That was the first time anyone ever realized that." He paused again and added, "And I think that includes me."
>
> (Goldberg, 1978, p. 271)

Wow! Nobody ever described anything like *that* to me in graduate school. The Ornsteins explained the profound effect on the state of the self that this kind of empathic understanding has by stating, "Feeling understood is the adult equivalent of being held ... which results in firming up or consolidating the self" (P. Ornstein & Ornstein, 1996, p. 94).

The second example is from the 1984 book *Kohut's Legacy*, a collection of articles edited by Arnold Goldberg and Paul Stepansky. Anna Ornstein's chapter in that book (Ornstein, 1984) tells of a patient who constantly insisted she needed to confront him and forcefully overcome his defenses and resistances to expose his hidden thoughts and feelings. If you know anything about Anna Ornstein, you know that this is *not* how she operates; nor, of course, does any self psychologist. Anna beautifully goes on to describe how she explores and stays empathic to her patient's wish for these aggressive interventions on her part, even though he is describing a version of therapeutic action that is completely antithetical to what she believes. So this was another revelation and example for me of how to remain empathically attuned when someone tells you something you disagree with fundamentally.

Finally, there is an article in the same book (Goldberg & Stepansky, 1984) by Brandchaft and Stolorow titled, "A Current Perspective on Difficult Patients." For me this was probably the most transformative thing I ever read in self psychology. First, it introduced me to intersubjectivity theory. Second, it offered me a radically different way from what I'd been taught for both how to understand and how to respond to severe psychopathology and borderline states. Echoing the emphasis on context that runs through our theory to this day, Brandchaft and Stolorow explained that when understandings and interventions isolate symptomatology from its intersubjective context, they risk rupture of the therapeutic relationship and an iatrogenic exacerbation of the symptoms. The article ends with a discussion of aggression and a passionately stated disagreement with the then-prevailing view that excessive aggression was the etiological bedrock of borderline and narcissistic pathology. In their words,

> Such excessive aggression is the inevitable, unwitting consequence of a therapeutic approach which insists that certain arrested archaic needs and the archaic states of mind associated with them are in their essence pathological dependency on or hostility toward the analyst. A vulnerable patient revives his most personal, nuclear, and vital needs in the relationship to the analyst. When these are misunderstood and misconstrued, and once again the patient is required to see his experiences from another's viewpoint when he so desperately longs for someone to see them from his own, it is not surprising that intense rage, destructiveness, and distrust may follow.
>
> (Brandchaft & Stolorow, 1984, p. 113)

I never saw people with borderline personality organizations the same way again after reading that. And of course, I learned that the concepts of intersubjectivity, context, co-creation and mutual influence are crucial for understanding all human behavior, not just borderline phenomena.

So what did *you* read that opened your eyes in a new way? I encourage you to think about it, and perhaps chat about it with your colleagues. What have you read lately? I'm describing my earliest experiences of this, but it never stops. I subsequently got so much from reading Brandchaft, more Stolorow, Teicholz, Geist and too many others to name. My most recent "aha" moment was reading a discussion by Estelle Shane of a case by Paolo Stramba-Badiale, just in (what was then) the most recent issue of *Psychoanalytic Inquiry* (Shane, 2014). Estelle explicated Edelman's concept of memory, primary and higher order consciousness as a way to explain the experience and mechanism of dissociation and flashback states. Reading it, I suddenly understood, in a way I'd never thought about, why a patient of mine was having so much trouble changing. It was so helpful. Our development that comes from reading never stops.

Not everyone has the good fortune of finding a mentor like Miriam Elson. But anyone can go to a self psychology conference, a local program or a web-based seminar. The international self psychology conferences have been a fertile ground of mentors and teachers for me. I have learned as much going to them each year as I have from any of the other strands in my self psychology tapestry. Years ago a study group member of mine attending her first self psychology conference said, "I feel like I have been studying a foreign language in a language laboratory and I have suddenly traveled to the country where they speak the language." The twinship experience of being surrounded by like-minded others, the opportunity to listen to the people who wrote what you've been reading, to find idealized teachers and to be so immersed in a set of ideas for three or four days can have a huge impact. The dialogue and comments of co-participants in post-panel discussion groups and other formal and informal exchanges have also been an important source of stimulation and learning for me—certainly not every time, but some of the most useful things I've heard, and in fact often incorporated into my own lectures, have been from random, spontaneous comments made in a discussion or a response to a question. The tremendous value of dialogue with colleagues is similarly what makes study groups such an important source of professional development for many people. In terms of our conferences, the opportunity to form friendships with people throughout the world is an added, wonderful bonus.

At the self psychology meetings I have met a number of people through whom continued dialogue has helped and fostered my professional development in a variety of ways. Among other things, conferences like that are networking opportunities, a chance to make contact with colleagues who may share your particular interests or more senior people who might later guide your writing, consult on your clinical work or invite you to present or coauthor an article. Many of our self psychology all-stars attend these meetings. Believe me, you can find people there who can help you bump up your game.

Having talked about reading, mentors and conferences as important vectors of professional development, I want to turn now to the experience of personal therapy by describing three moments in my work with Paul Tolpin. I had had some very good psychodynamic supervisors during my training, albeit with a more classical orientation. And I had earlier, in my 20s, seen a very good therapist, a training analyst even. But none of that enabled me to understand what deep empathic immersion really means until my experience with Paul.

Fairly early in the process, one day I discounted something he was saying with the words, "But it's not like this is a *real* relationship. I mean it's not like we go to the movies together or anything." Without the slightest hesitation, Paul responded, "But of course we do! We go to the interior movies together." So few words needed to convey both where I needed to focus and how ready he was to join me there. "Oh," I said, suddenly filled with his warmth.

Another day, for reasons I can no longer remember, I felt like I wasn't shouldering my share of something or other and was leaning on others too much. So I said, with a fair degree of self-contempt, "I feel like a leech!" Paul immediately yet rather gently protested, "But even a leech has to eat, in the only way it knows how." Such radical acceptance. And I leave thinking, "I can't believe this. He can even be empathic to a leech!"

In retrospect, of course, I can more clearly understand that he was saying if I had another way of operating, I'd be doing it. Paul always, always kept his ear to the forward edge, the positive, growth-seeking reason for anything defensive, dysfunctional or disruptive, and the tendril of health hidden in it.[3]

But the one that made the most indelible impression on me, when it comes to a depth of being immersed in another's subjective experience, is the day Paul told me it would be better for me if he died. I assure you he had no death wish. It happened like this. One day Paul was late coming to meet me in his waiting room. This was atypical. My mind moved through a series of possible explanations for it, which I shared with him as we finally started the session. I said,

> At first I thought you probably were running over with a patient and I didn't think much of it. Then it seemed too long and I thought maybe you got distracted and lost track of time. After a while I started wondering if you had forgotten me, maybe even didn't really want to see me, were actually sick of me or would rather be doing something else. I stayed with that for a while and then I started thinking maybe you died and were just dead in there and that's why you weren't coming.

At this point, Paul suddenly interrupted me and said, with considerable enthusiasm, "Oh, but that would be so much better!" Later I thought, does his empathy know no bounds? Can he be so immersed in my experience that he can, that instantly, convey an understanding that what would be terrible for him (in fact fatal) would be a relief to me, because then I would know it wasn't personal? I was flabbergasted by the steadfastness with which he could stay with my internal world, which then transformed a rupture into a moment of meeting (Stern et al., 1998). It was also a vivid experience of a central tenet of self psychology: that we look for what a patient is doing right, not wrong, and what her behavior expresses, rather than what it distorts or defends against. Now I knew that. I had read all the articles that say that. But I knew it in my head, not in my gut; I knew it superficially, not in depth—a huge difference.

As a postscript, I would add that Paul did eventually ask me why I hadn't rung the bell to let him know I was waiting. I didn't say a word. I just shrugged and gave him a look that I'm sure conveyed something like, "Seriously?" Again, without needing any further input from me, he answered his own question with, "Of course, because you wanted me to remember."

No matter how much I ever might have read or how many conferences I attended, I don't know whether I ever truly could have understood self psychology without the experience of my relationships with Paul Tolpin and Miriam Elson. These experiences in turn informed my work as a supervisor, underscoring the necessity of trainees having a lived experience of empathy rather than just reading or hearing about it.

In our effort to teach, we can forget this, as I did in the following situation.[4] I was supervising a psychology intern who came with a generally cognitive/behavioral orientation to psychotherapy. He had approached me with an avowed interest in learning about self psychology. But after months of trying to help him understand how to assume a more empathic vantage point in relation to his patients' experience, I found him still operating mainly via a highly directive, rational and educative mode of talking with them. Eventually, in response to his ceaseless activity, I retreated to a state of what Brightman (1984) called "fatigued resignation."

It then happened that the supervisee experienced a tragedy in his family: the sudden, accidental death of a sibling. In our first supervisory meeting after his return, I expressed my condolences and inquired how he was. In response, he spent the rest of the session talking entirely about this event. I listened intently during this conversation and said very little, but felt intensely "with" him—perhaps in that particular right-brain-to-right-brain way we think about these days. The next week he returned to talking about his cases as usual in our meeting.

However, the week after that he brought a case into supervision and told me how for the first time it made sense to him to just sit with his patient and listen to him. "I suddenly realized maybe I had something to offer by doing that," he said. He then told me about his experience of our previous conversation about his family. "I never had an experience quite like that. When you spoke, *I felt like your breath came through me* ... like you not only knew how I felt but *felt* how I felt." This profound experience of empathy made a dramatic impression on him. Despite my previous attempts to help him adopt a more empathic stance, he needed to experience it as something of value before he could in turn provide a similar experience to his patients.

Unsurprisingly, this marked a turning point in our supervision. At the end of the training year, as we reviewed our history together and all the unproductive recycling in the same patterns we had done before this breakthrough, he said to me, "Yeah, what took you so long?" And he was right. After initial, failed attempts at trying to understand his experience, I had eventually met his endless harangues of his patients with harangues of my own about not making harangues.

This is reminiscent of Sloan's (1986) conclusion that trying to impart what he called all his "pent up wisdom" about empathy to his psychiatric residents only resulted in their similarly assuming "authoritatively knowledgeable and directive roles" (p. 189) with their own patients. He also provided a nice description of the alternative:

> The more I was able to ... acknowledge, appreciate ... or place in a larger context something of value in what my residents experienced as naturally and authentically *their own* (even when very different from mine), the more confident and competent they became with their patients ... At the same time, they seemed to become more capable of adopting an empathic vantage point with their patients, which in turn brought more usable material into supervision. In short, they learned to listen best by having someone listen to them.
>
> (p. 190)

Returning to my example, I certainly don't think that a single experience transforms personality. But I do believe there are moments of meeting that in and of themselves are transformative, as I believe the particular experience I described was for this supervisee.

I would like to share one last vignette from my experience as a supervisor. This one is from early in my career and demonstrates what happens when you don't know anything about self psychology. I share it for two reasons. First, I like to teach from some of my more spectacular failures—it seems to really make people feel good—and this is one of my all-time favorites, a real doozy. Second, I promised in the beginning to try to be at least a little funny, and I feel I haven't quite come through enough yet on that count. This story, for some reason, has a tendency to make people laugh.

> I am supervising a third-year medical student in his psychiatry rotation. He has a passive-aggressive female patient, toward whom he is feeling very angry because she isn't changing. He vents his anger at the patient, just blasts her. She responds by oversleeping for a noon session the following week. In supervision I try to help him recognize his hostile feelings and behavior toward the patient. He resists this strongly. He then forgets his next supervisory session, recapitulating his patient's passive-aggressive behavior with his own supervisor. I'm excited. I figure now he'll get it. So I try to interpret his acting out with me and anger at me for having confronted him with his anger at the patient. He again resists strongly, refusing to own any such feelings, and essentially conveying that he thinks I'm talking some kind of psychobabble. So what do you suppose happens next? In a profoundly embarrassing development, I forget our next supervisory session, now passive-aggressively acting out my own anger and frustration with the student, whom I cannot get through to. We thus came full circle, with every dyad (patient to therapist, therapist to supervisor, and finally supervisor to therapist) doing exactly the same thing in the same way. As one set of authors writing about parallel process put it, the unconscious has a "disregard for time, place, or seniority" (Gediman & Wolkenfeld, 1980, p. 253).

Operating without a theory that would have directed me to inner experience, I had repeated the student's error of being interpretive, confrontational and angry, rather than trying to understand what was going on for him. It is likely that his patient was making him feel frustrated, helpless and inadequate, but I simply left him in the lurch with these or any other feelings she might have been evoking in him. This vignette underscores once again that the process we want our students to use with their patients is one we must also offer to them.

Now, before wrapping all this up, I want to comment on what perhaps has sounded like a rather narrow focus here in terms of therapeutic action. I realize, of course, that there is more to self psychology than empathic understanding, whether framed in terms of the resolution of selfobject transference, illumination and transformation of unconscious organizing principles, the integration and transformation of affect or the numerous other ways we have of conceptualizing and describing the therapeutic endeavor. Also, our contemporary focus on context, mutual influence and co-construction necessitates that the therapist be aware of, open to and able to manage his or her own affective and subjective experience, and to recognize its impact on the treatment (e.g., Teicholz, 2014). I haven't spoken to any of that. I've focused on empathy because, no matter how our theories evolve, I think it remains at the heart of them. It is also, in my experience, one of the hardest things to learn to do consistently and well.

The idea of something constant at the core while also changing is poignantly expressed in a poem I'm very fond of. It is called "The Layers" and was written by Stanley Kunitz, an American poet laureate, when he was 80 years old (Kunitz, 2005). In the first verse, he describes how after walking through many different lives, his own and others, he may not be who he was, yet his life maintains an abiding principle of being from which he strives not to stray. In the last verse, he says he is not done with his changes, that his next chapter of transformation is undoubtedly already written, though he is not yet able to decipher what it will be.

So it is with the self and with our theories: Something remains central and continuous, even as both—self and theory—continue to grow, transform and change.

So, let me now try to pull this all together by way of conclusion. Planning these words originally for delivery in the ancient city of Jerusalem, so important to at least three of the world's great religions, brings me back to the biblical text I mentioned in the beginning. I return to Abraham, common ancestor, through Ishmael and Isaac, of both Muslims and Jews. Abraham's God commands him not only *lech lecha*, go forth on this journey, but in the next verse, "*vehyay b'racha*," be a blessing. I think this means give back, be a blessing to others, help the people behind you on their journey. In our context, that might mean become a conference welcomer, an IAPSP committee member or chair, a teacher, a supervisor, or mentor, a presenter or writer, or even just someone who listens with profound depth to another human being. Offer lower-cost treatment, if you can, to a junior member of our field, so he or she will know what it *feels* like to have the experience of being in the care of a self psychologist.

L'dor v'dor, from generation to generation. Heinz Kohut analyzed Paul Tolpin. Paul Tolpin analyzed me and gave me the experience of a self psychological treatment. Miriam Elson wrote a book that opened the gates of self psychology theory and writings to me. With her encouragement, I wrote an article on brief treatment that tried to clarify core concepts in a similarly accessible way. Miriam nurtured and mentored me professionally, and I, in turn, have tried to nurture and mentor a number of others. *L'dor v'dor*, from generation to generation, I implore you: *vehyay b'racha*, be a blessing, and give back. Those of you reading this now, along with many others of our founders and leaders, have so much to offer. Thank you.

Notes

1 Historically, the Kohut Memorial Lecture is given at the end of a luncheon.
2 Tolpin was part of the original, small group of Chicago analysts with whom Kohut shared and discussed early versions of his works.
3 See Tolpin (2002) for a fuller discussion of the concept of the forward edge.
4 For a complete description of this and similar vignettes, see Gardner (1995).

References

Beebe, B., & Lachmann, F. (1994). Representation and internalization in infancy: Three principles of salience. *Psychoanalytic Psychology, 11*, 127–165.

Brandchaft, B., & Stolorow, R. (1984). A current perspective on difficult patients. In A. Goldberg & P. Stepansky (Eds.), *Kohut's legacy* (pp. 93–115). Hillsdale, NJ: Analytic Press.

Brightman, B. (1984). Narcissistic issues in the training experience of the psychotherapist. *International Journal of Psychoanalytic Psychotherapy, 10*, 293–317.

Elson, M. (1986). *Self psychology in clinical social work*. New York, NY: W.W. Norton & Company.

Gardner, J. (1995). Supervision of trainees: Tending the professional self. *Clinical Social Work Journal, 23*, 271–286.

Gardner, J. (2015). Journeys and generations: Tending the professional self. *Psychoanalysis, Self and Context, 10*, 408–420.

Gediman, H., & Wolkenfeld, F. (1980). The parallelism phenomenon in psychoanalysis and supervision: Its reconsideration as a triadic system. *Psychoanalytic Quarterly, 49*, 234–255.

Goldberg, A. (1978). *The psychology of the self: A casebook.* New York, NY: International Universities Press.

Goldberg, A., & Stepansky, P. (Eds.). (1984). *Kohut's legacy.* Hillsdale, NJ: Analytic Press.

Kohut, H. (1971). *The analysis of the self.* New York, NY: International Universities Press.

Kohut, H. (1977). *The restoration of the self.* New York, NY: International Universities Press.

Kohut, H. (1984). *How does analysis cure?* Chicago, IL: University of Chicago Press.

Kunitz, S. (2005). *The wild braid: A poet reflects on a century in the garden.* New York: W.W. Norton & Company.

Ornstein, A. (1984). Psychoanalytic psychotherapy: A contemporary perspective. In A. Goldberg & P. Stepansky (Eds.), *Kohut's legacy* (pp. 171–181). Hillsdale, NJ: Analytic Press.

Ornstein, P., & Ornstein, A. (1996). I. Some general principles of psychoanalytic psychotherapy: A self-psychological perspective. In L. Lifson (Ed.), *Understanding therapeutic action: Psychodynamic concepts of cure* (pp. 87–101). Hillsdale, NJ: The Analytic Press.

Shane, E. (2014). Explaining trauma in highly traumatized patients: A brain-based psychoanalytic perspective. *Psychoanalytic Inquiry, 34,* 315–321.

Sloan, J. (1986). The empathic vantage point in supervision. In A. Goldberg (Ed.), *Progress in self psychology* (Vol. 2, pp. 188–211). New York, NY: Guilford Press.

Socarides, D., & Stolorow, R. (1984–1985). Affects and selfobjects. *The Annual of Psychoanalysis, 12/13,* 105–119.

Stern, D., Sander, L., Nahum, J., Harrison, A., Lyons-Ruth, K., Morgan, A., Bruschweilerstern, N., & Tronick, E. (1998). Non-interpretive mechanisms in psychoanalytic therapy: The "something more" than interpretation. *International Journal of Psychoanalysis, 79,* 903–921.

Teicholz, J. (2014). Treating trauma: The analyst's own affect regulation and expression. *Psychoanalytic Inquiry, 34,* 364–379.

Tolpin, M. (2002). Doing psychoanalysis of normal development: Forward edge transferences. *Progress in Self Psychology, 18,* 167–190.

Winnicott, D.W. (1965). *The maturational processes and the facilitating environment.* New York, NY: International Universities Press.

Wolf, E.S. (1988). *Treating the self: elements of clinical self psychology.* New York, NY: Guilford Press.

Index

adaptations, adaptive responses 5, 52–56, 108, 109, 113n3, 128
adolescents, young adults 31, 33, 66
affective resonance 80, 82
affirmation, affirming responsiveness 12, 28, 29, 30, 60, 61, 80, 92–93
agency 107, 112–115, 118, 131, 136–138; self-agency 106–113, 131 (*see also under own heading*); sense of 106, 108–109, 111–113
aggression 81, 117, 149
alter-ego experiences 38
ambitions 24–26, 31, 37, 58, 85, 92
American Psychological Association (APA) 3
Annual Conference on the Psychology of the Self (2006) 100
Atwood, George E. 119, 134, 135
Axis II personality disorders 4, 7

Bacal, Howard A. 42, 87
Balint, P. 32n2, 54
Bacal, H. 13, 41, 87
Basch, Michael F. 42, 44, 46–47, 48, 57–59, 63, 73n2, 107, 118, 127
bi-directionality / bi-directional influences 117, 118, 135
borderline patients, borderline states 3, 4, 62, 149
Brandchaft, Bernard 108, 149
brief focal psychotherapy 55
brief psychotherapy treatment 8–32, 36–74; as appropriate self psychology application 8, 9, 36; case examples: Jim 17–26, 26–29, 31, 32; communication needs 31, 42; course correction 69–70; empathic interpretations of selfobject experience 65–69; focus 16–17,

28–29, 32, 49–50; mutative moments 70–71; patient selection, patient suitability 31–32, 45–48; planning 48–49; precipitating events 61–65; The Self, state of 50–65 (*see also under own heading*); as self psychology practice 14–17, 31, 43–45; symptoms, symptomatic behaviors/expressions 5, 29–31, 49, 50–52 (*see also under own heading*); termination, object/selfobject loss 71–72; therapist mindset 29–30
Brightman, B. 79, 147, 152

case examples and vignettes: empathic communication and responsiveness, 138–140; empathic understanding 148; Jim (brief psychotherapy) 43–55, 57; self-agency (David) 111–112, 113; supervision, supervisory relationship 83–84, 88–89, 90–92, 139–140, 154
Chernus, L. 15–16, 43–44
child, childhood development: case examples: David 108 / Jim 23–24, 27; early selfobject milieu, adequacy 38; efficacy selfobject experience 107; empathic parent response 38, 131; empathic responsiveness need 4, 131; experience of the grandiose self, early expansiveness 9, 11; idealized parent imago 10, 37; magnets for development, parent–child 101, 118–119; misattunement, trauma 107–108, 110, 128; motivational primacy of self experience 10, 38; parent's self strengthening, self objects 88, 101; self-agency development 106–107, 131; self-esteem development 11
Contorer, Betty 32n2